# Health and Medicine
# in the Methodist Tradition

# Health/Medicine and the Faith Traditions

## Edited by Martin E. Marty and Kenneth L. Vaux

*Health/Medicine and the Faith Traditions*
explores the ways in which major religions
relate to the questions of human well-being.
It issues from Project Ten, an interfaith program
of The Park Ridge Center, An Institute for the Study of
Health, Faith, and Ethics.

James P. Wind, Director of Research and Publications

The Park Ridge Center
is part of the Lutheran General Health Care System,
Park Ridge, Illinois.

# Health and Medicine in the Methodist Tradition

## JOURNEY TOWARD WHOLENESS

E. Brooks Holifield

Crossroad · New York

1986
The Crossoad Publishing Company
370 Lexington Ave, New York, N.Y. 10017

*Library of Congress Cataloging in Publication Data*

Holified, E. Brooks
Health and medicine in the Methodist tradition.

(Health/Medicine and the faith traditions)
Bibliograpy: p.
1. Health—Religious aspects—Methodist Church.
2. Medicine—Religious aspects—Methodist Church.
3. Methodist Church—Doctrines. I. Title. II. Series.
[DNLM: 1. Pastoral Care. 2. Religion and Medicine.
3. Religion and Psychology. W 50 H732h]
BX8349.H4H65 1986      261.5'6      86-16770
ISBN 0-8245-0792-4

*To my mother*

# Contents

# Foreword

One could make the case that John Wesley was the true Protestant genius between the sixteenth-century Reformation and our day. Similarly, the Wesleyan and Methodist movements were the Western religious forces that first and best caught on to what modernity involved for spiritual and churchly life.

These are large claims. Martin Luther and John Calvin and other Reformers everyone knows, whether religious or not. John Wesley, it would seem, only Wesleyans and Methodists, if even *they*, would know and be able to locate. But the global importance of John Wesley and his followers stems from their perception of modernity's demand that faith be made portable. On the whole, Catholic and early Protestant Europe continued to act as if "faith came with the territory," as if religion passed through the genes to new generations. They assumed that all in a certain region or country should adopt the faith of their rulers. Wesley and the evangelists, revivalists, and awakeners at his side and in his train spotted something new. They recognized the democratic and mobile human being of the English industrial city and the American frontier. The church had to go out to find such people, to attract their attention, to fire them up, to get them to "decide" for God, to seek the way of grace and perfection. And then it had to form new communities of care, fervent if voluntary.

Wesley in a sense is a symbolic name for all those field preachers and chapel builders, those riders of boats and horses who went out to find the people and give Christianity a new impetus; "the world is my parish!" was a typical depiction of their scope. Yet he also deserves priority for his personal genius as a reformer within Anglicanism who kept what he could of the past and as a reluctant founder of a new movement who sobersidedly allowed for new excitements.

For a century or two Methodism was one of the most successful movements in Western Christendom. Until recently it was the largest Protestant group in the United States (it has now yielded place to Southern Baptists).

Until less recently it was the most lively non-established Protestant church in England, although slippage there has been drastic and the yielding has been more to secular forces than to another church. Was Methodism too adapted to one stage of modernity and thus unable to pioneer in postmodern times, when more rigid and extravagant movements took over? This is not the place to chronicle declines in Methodism. There are still well over 10 million members in the United States. These people, called Wesleyan or Methodist, have needs for health and well-being, some of which have been met or could be met out of resources in their distinctive tradition. What is more, that tradition, whose founder himself was uncommonly interested in health and healing and care, has insights, practices, and suggestions that can be helpful as well to non-Wesleyans or non-Methodists.

The terms *Wesleyan* and *Methodist*, which I have found myself sliding between, have slightly different nuances. In the most proper sense, Holifield speaks of the Wesleyan tradition. But who in today's America would know what to do with that? Some might know of universities in West Virginia or Nebraska or South Dakota that had *Wesleyan* in their title. What else?

Reference books will not give readers an idea of the weight of this subject. The Chicago Yellow Pages, for example, lists only five small congregations under the heading "Churches—Wesleyan, The," and one of them does not even use the name. The *Yearbook of American and Canadian Churches 1985* puts them in the company of 1,722 congregations and 107,672 members. The *World Christian Encyclopedia* estimates that there are 22,190 separate Christian bodies in the world, so it is not likely that a handful of Wesleyan-named ones will press themselves on the consciousness of Christians or others.

One would expect proud Methodists to be custodians of the Wesleyan tradition. A personal illustration will suggest that they are not. In 1983, the five hundredth birthday of Luther coincided with the two hundredth anniversary of American Methodism. That fall I shared a platform with Albert C. Outler, Methodist historian-theologian supreme, at a United Methodist ministers' week at Duke University. After the two of us had lectured on our assigned subjects, we were asked to "switch" informally for a question period. In my short statement I attempted to show how American Methodism could move ahead if it revisited and developed its roots in Wesley. Outler, with courteous smile, commented that until then he had respected this Lutheran historian, but that day I failed him. "Marty is so naive as to think that American Methodism knows about its founder John Wesley."

Outler may have blended mild cynicism, well-earned weariness, and the hope that he could chide his fellow-believers into awareness. The roots are, for many, thin and forgotten. Yet while the churches that derive from his witness may not know much about him, much of what he stood for influenced their attitudes and outlook and helps shape many who have never heard of him.

Professor Holifield's work details exactly how. I can, however, offer a semi-outsider's view. As already noted, between the era of Luther and Calvin, and our time, he represents as individual and as symbol the genius of adaptation to modernity. Philosopher Alfred North Whitehead scored the movement for failing to appeal to any "great intellectual construction explanatory of its modes of understanding" and for having begun by "instinct" to waver in its appeal to constructive reason. Yet he decided that "it may have chosen the better way" overall. For in England and America, among working people and pioneers, the Wesleyans "brought hope, fear, emotional release, spiritual insight," and some humanitarianism. H. Richard Niebuhr has identified Wesley, along with Pope Gregory the Great and Martin Luther, as a pivotal figure in pastoral care. There are several reasons to pursue his pioneering impulses.

First, this modern—no enemy of science and a friend of medicine—was not afraid of modernity. While we may chuckle at some of the Wesleyan nostrums and bizarre medical theories, they were not far off the mark of the best scientific efforts of his time. And they did show a passionate regard for humans in their suffering, a warm concern for their bodies, and a sense that he and his workers must care and cure not only in the realm of soul-saving, their chosen sphere, but also in the search for temporal well-being. That tradition has not been exhausted. It is, in fact, only now being recovered widely.

Second, Wesley knew the importance of social relations in the search for well-being. He provided classes, patterns of discipline, motives for self-expression that have led one modern Methodist, Thomas Oden, to argue at book length that most of what is worthwhile in contemporary group therapy is consistent with and in some ways flows from Wesley's understanding that people need support of other people, and also that they like to supply it.

To these two I would add a theme emphasized by Holifield. Wesley's doctrine of holiness and sanctification involved a *journey* toward wholeness. One still senses a dynamism in these old Wesley texts: it is hard to picture him talking about a "state" of health or a "condition" of well-being, for these imply fulfillment and stasis. No, in language that contemporaries can well understand, he addressed what pilgrims, restless ones, seekers, are about. The metaphor of a spiritual journey has come back into personal life along with the image of the "pilgrim church" that is prominent in Catholic and Protestant life alike and that has parallels in other religions.

Wesley also respected the values of pluralism. Today's United Methodist bearers of the Wesleyan tradition both encourage pluralism and fear that it may be so conceived as to create problems, such as the toleration of license or the blurring of identities. Yet the alternatives Wesley confronted were worse, and his sense of trust in God and others, his promotion of choice and development of freedom assured that the Wesleyan tradition was not to be narrow, confining, easily defined. Holifield shows how from Richard Allen to James Cone the Methodist movement made room for blacks, and in the deaconess movement and in other ways, for women. Methodism has no single consistent binding theology, but there is a "feel" for Methodist rightness; it has a character, some distinctives.

Finally, the Wesleyan tradition carries a positive virus to change the world. The religions of the West as Wesley knew them tended to be passive, part of the status quo. He was hardly a revolutionary, though some prominent historians have argued that he bought off discontent and channeled energies so that England was spared a shooting revolution. Be that as it may, he believed that churches and church people had to promote well-being wherever they were. Drinkers, they became temperance people when they saw destruction of families through uncontrolled drinking. They built hospitals, worked for just laws, established universities, promoted scientific study of medicine and up-to-date study of theology.

Theology, yes. Methodism does not often get credit for that. Yet a reader of Holifield is likely to notice many congenial names in medical ethics and humane theology. Paul Ramsey is a Methodist layman; Stanley Hauerwas shares the tradition. Both have applied their learning to questions of morality and medicine. Theologians of years ago like Edgar S. Brightman and Borden Parker Bowne share pages here with Schubert Ogden and John Cobb, current theological bearers of the tradition. Many pioneers in the pastoral counseling field—Russell Dicks and Carroll Wise or, in England, Leslie Weatherhead—were encouraged in this tradition.

The Wesleyan tradition does not begin with and certainly did not end with John Wesley. His busy followers and colleagues caught that positive virus to change the world, including the diseased bodies of people in need; to reform the world, beginning with the half-faithful minds of their contemporaries. They kept inventing and patenting, as it were, therapies and patterns to help others make a modern journey toward wholeness. This book is a road map that will help many find how far they have come on that journey, whether they are lost, and how to move on to a new understanding and vantage. One need not be a Methodist, a Nazarene, a Pentecostal, a Holiness person to share the need for wholeness or to profit from the resources Professor Holifield has helped make available.

MARTIN E. MARTY

# Introduction

John Wesley, the founder of the Methodist movement, would have relished the opportunity to write this volume. He recognized the power of religious traditions, and he thought that issues of health and medicine were profoundly interwoven into the texture of religious faith. All ten themes that have concerned Project X—healing and well-being, suffering and madness, passages and sexuality, dying and caring, morality and dignity—were among the topics that Wesley believed should interest Christians.

Wesley was no systematic theologian, and he left us no single body of systematic reflection on health and medicine. If he had, we probably would view it somewhat as we now view his popular little manual of medical prescriptions: it would be quaint, and of interest to antiquarians, but too firmly rooted in the eighteenth century to be of much use in the twentieth. Hence the theologian who wishes to understand Wesley's legacy must undertake not only a historical task but also a constructive one.

The task of this volume is partly historical: the recovery of what Wesley and Methodists have said about medicine and health. But I have attempted to interpret those reflections by locating them within a particular style of theological discourse. If I am successful, the broad theological patterns that shape the book will be judged as both faithful to Wesley's larger vision and consistent with the spirit of later theological reflection among Methodists.

The metaphor of journeying aptly captures the spirit of Methodist theology, for Wesley viewed theology as a practical endeavor which had as its aim the guidance of the Christian life. Theological notions were for Wesley and for later Methodists not so much instruments of a speculative science as guideposts for the Christian who wanted to remain faithfully within the "way of salvation," or the way of love.

The polarities outlined in the following chapters, though formulated more systematically than Wesley himself attempted, help to show how the Wesleyan understanding of theology might inform a modern Methodist sensibility. The polarities of health and healing, holiness and happiness, penalty and promise, love and law, restraint and responsibility, and possibility and limit provide a way of establishing boundaries; they mark the way of a journey. They are not to be construed as opposites or as mutually exclusive extremes. Each member of each pair both checks and enriches the other.

Wesley was not inclined to think in disjunctions—either health or healing, either holiness or happiness, either penalty or promise. He preferred the conjunctions—both health and healing, both holiness and happiness, both penalty and promise. But the conjunctions also embodied a certain tension precluding any fixed and final synthesis. At its best the Methodist tradition has honored the tension, shying away from claims to finality and remaining aware that we see only as through a mirror darkly.

My construction of the polarities is an attempt to interpret the Methodist tradition, not to render any classic Methodist statement. But the theological interpretation presented here is tied closely to the Wesleyan heritage, and therefore each chapter begins with the eighteenth-century origins of the tradition. The narrative form of the chapters combines historical and theological reflection; this seems much more in keeping with the Methodist tradition than would be a sharper systematic outline, and the narrative style coincides appropriately with the metaphor of the journey. I have chosen to concentrate not on institutional achievements or on the social history of Methodism but on ideas and themes that might provide critical insights into persistent issues. It is not the purpose of the Project X series to sponsor denominational pride, and though I trust I have not ignored Methodist accomplishments, I hope I have avoided the temptation to make them the centerpiece of the narrative.

The Methodist tradition was not the only fruit of the eighteenth-century Wesleyan movement in England: "holiness" and Pentecostal churches join the larger Methodist groups in tracing their roots to the theology and ministry of John Wesley. The Methodist tradition, however, is itself so complex that the effort to include other Wesleyan groups in the story would have severely burdened an already complicated account. In any case, the editors of the Project X series plan to offer more extended coverage to holiness and Pentecostal traditions within the covers of another book in the series.

The Methodist movement began in the eighteenth century as a religious revival within the Church of England, directed mainly to the poor and outcast. Its founder was an Anglican priest who ventured to preach in the open fields to the colliers and laborers of England, Scotland, and Wales. Separate Methodist churches began to emerge in America in 1784 when Wesley's followers decided, despite his ambivalence, to form a communion outside the boundaries of Anglicanism. By the time Wesley died in 1791, his followers in England were moving gradually toward a similar decision.

Within a century of Wesley's death, Methodists formed the largest Protestant group in the United States, presented a significant alternative to Anglicanism in England, and attracted adherents in smaller numbers throughout Europe, Asia, South America, and Africa. In the late nineteenth century, they retained much of their earlier revivalist fervor, but they also displayed a new sense of liturgical decorum, a cautious curiosity about the new theologies of the day, a growing preference for an educated ministry, and a conspicuous interest in social reforms.

Methodists in the late twentieth century, especially in the United States, tend often to identify themselves by either a plaintive or a proud reference to their *pluralism*. The term refers to the diversity of Methodist theological views, the variety of Methodist liturgical styles, and the manifold forms of Methodist piety. That pluralism creates problems for the historian trying to define a Methodist *tradition*, so the first chapter, which deals chiefly with the links between Wesley's theology and his views about health and medicine, also addresses the question of what it might mean to speak of an enduring Methodist heritage.

For criticisms of the first draft of this manuscript, I am indebted especially to James Wind, Albert Outler, Stephen Stein, and Paul Thigpen. My students at Emory University also proved to be insightful critics of early formulations. For all their suggestions I am grateful, even while knowing they will be disappointed that I failed to make better use of them.

# Part I

# JOURNEY

# · 1 ·

# Wesley and His Tradition

More than once John Wesley described himself as a "man of just one book," a man determined "to study (comparatively) no book but the Bible." More than once he referred to himself as "a creature of a day, passing through life as an arrow shot through the air," and therefore interested only in one thing—"the way to heaven." He insisted that men and women were sent into the world for "one sole end, and for no other, to prepare for eternity." More than once, moreover, he defined his task and the task of his followers as simply the pursuit of "holiness of heart and life," and it became a commonplace of later Methodists that their grand object was to "spread scriptural holiness" throughout the land. Here, surely, was a man whose eyes were fixed on the prospect of salvation in another world, not on the promise of health and healing in this one.[1]

Yet Wesley the man of one book also read more than a thousand other books by more than a thousand authors; he edited dozens of books on a myriad of topics, including several on health and medicine; and he took great satisfaction in the popularity of his own medical guidebook, *Primitive Physick*, which he urged his preachers to recommend to their congregations. "It is a great pity," he once wrote, "that any Methodist should be without [it]."[2] Wesley the creature of a day, preparing himself and others for eternal salvation, had members of his societies visit the sick every other day and provide for their temporal needs. And Wesley the evangelist, spreading scriptural holiness throughout the land, also established medical dispensaries in English cities for diagnosis and treatment of the sick.

Wesley believed that even the name *Methodist*, by which he and his followers were known, contained an oblique reference to the practice of medicine. When a fellow student at Oxford satirized the order and regularity of behavior in Wesley's small Holy Club by suggesting that "we have got a new sect of Methodists," Wesley assumed that the satirist was "alluding

3

to a sect of physicians who began to flourish at Rome about the time of Nero, and continued for several ages."[3] Wesley never made much of the allusion, but in retrospect it seems oddly appropriate.

Where does one find the inner link between Wesley the pilgrim and Wesley the physician? How did he understand the relationship between the one book, the Scripture, with its proclamations about the law and the gospel, and the medical book, with its prescriptions for agues and apoplexy? Is it possible to clarify Wesley's interest in medicine and health by locating it within his broader theological vision?

Because Wesley founded an enduring religious tradition, such questions lead us quickly beyond mere antiquarian curiosity. In trying to answer them, one encounters larger issues, not simply about Wesley but also about the traditions which flowed from his movement. How has the Methodist tradition linked Wesley the pilgrim and Wesley the physician? How has it understood the relationship between faith and therapy? Can one speak meaningfully about a Methodist perspective on health and medicine? The argument of this book is that it does make sense to talk about a Methodist tradition, that the tradition has addressed issues of medicine and health since its inception, and that such a tradition can still illumine those issues.

## A METHODIST TRADITION?

The Methodist societies that John Wesley founded in eighteenth-century England have developed into a vast family of churches with over 38 million members throughout the world. The largest of those churches, the United Methodist Church, located chiefly in the United States, has about 10 million members; the African Methodist Episcopal Church, also an American body, has over 2 million; the African Methodist Episcopal Zion Church has more than a million; the English Methodist Church more than eight hundred thousand. And Methodist congregations carry on the tradition from Korea to Ghana, from Germany to Australia, from Argentina to Kenya. Clearly one can speak meaningfully of Methodist traditions.

But are they Wesleyan? Do they remain in continuity with the eighteenth-century English revival in which John Wesley guided and nurtured his "People called Methodists"? The American Methodist theologians who gathered in 1972 at the General Conference of the United Methodist Church acknowledged their sense of a "bewildering spectrum of doctrinal diversity" within their denomination. "Somewhere in the United Methodist Church," they said, "there is somebody urging every kind of theology still alive and not a few that are dead." A recent historian of Christian doctrine, trying explicitly to understand "theology in the Wesleyan tradition," had finally to conclude that Methodist theological distinctiveness is, at best, "elusive." Even in England, where Methodists have often retained a stronger sense of continuity with Wesleyan doctrine, Methodist historians acknowledge that Methodism is often considered "more notable for its warmheartedness . . . than for the depth and width of its theological thought."[4]

The problem of defining a continuing Methodist tradition, and of clarifying its relationship to matters of health and medicine, is made more difficult by the fact that the Methodist churches have no binding confessional statement, no one document possessing the authority that Lutherans, for example, find in the Augsburg Confession. Wesley was wary of establishing a confessional test. Insisting that even his own collected sermons were to be accepted only insofar as they remained in accord with Scripture, he had no sympathy with anyone who defined Christian faith simply as "a string of opinions."[5]

For Wesley, right opinions were only a "slender part" of Christianity. To be sure, he was not as indifferent to doctrines as many of his later admirers wanted to suppose. He thought that certain affirmations had to be made. Christians could not surrender their convictions about the unique revelatory character of the Scripture, the unique status of Jesus Christ as both the eternal God and a particular man, and the unique gift of redemption in Christ through which God graciously offered salvation to the fallen creation. But he hoped to avoid entanglement in disputes about doctrinal niceties: "As to all opinions which do not strike at the root of Christianity, we think and let think."[6]

His wariness about divisive theological nit-picking formed the setting for Wesley's oft-cited statement of willingness to overlook differences of opinion: "Is thy heart right, as my heart is with thine? I ask no farther question. If it be, give me thy hand. For opinions, or terms, let us not destroy the work of God. Dost thou love and serve God? It is enough."[7] He was not issuing a general commendation of theological indifference, but his irenic temperament and his distaste for theological quibbling serve to compound the difficulties of the historian seeking to draw firm boundaries marking the Wesleyan tradition.

In the same way, Wesley's sensitivities to the breadth of the Christian tradition made him reluctant to overemphasize the distinctive doctrinal contours of his own movement. "From real Christians, of whatever denomination they be," he once said, "we earnestly desire not to be distinguished at all; not from any who sincerely follow after what they know they have not attained."[8] He believed that his preachers taught only the common, fundamental principles of Christianity and that those common principles cut across denominational boundaries. He had no interest in forming a new church—he remained within the Church of England—and he had no inclination to ferret out supposed doctrinal errors in other traditions.

It is ironic, then, that the problem of defining a Methodist tradition is now complicated further by historic divisions within that tradition itself. As late as 1930, there were at least nineteen denominations in the United States and at least three in England that bore the name Methodist and shared a heritage in Wesley's teaching. Subsequent mergers have reduced the proliferation, but Methodist churches still represent a startling array of liturgical and doctrinal traditions.

The diversity makes us ask what it means to speak of a tradition and of being formed by a tradition. It requires that we ask if disagreements can sometimes mask a common way of thinking about problems, a common style and inclination, that resists encapsulation in tight and rigid propositions yet maintains recognizable features. Hence we begin our quest for a Methodist tradition.

As a place of beginning, one might follow the lead of the theologians at the 1972 General Conference of the United Methodists in America and attempt to define a Methodist theological style. Those theologians drew on the Wesleyan standards—John Wesley's sermons, his *Explanatory Notes Upon the New Testament*, his abridged version of the Anglican Thirty-nine Articles of Religion—but tried to locate them within a "new context of interpretation." They sought to understand the norms to which Wesley appealed, and to grasp their implications for a contemporary restatement of the Wesleyan vision.

The result was an elaboration of what the Methodist theologian Albert Outler called the "Wesleyan quadrilateral." The quadrilateral was a statement and interpretation of the four theological criteria to which Wesley appealed as a Christian teacher. The primary source was *Scripture*, the unique testimony to God's self-disclosures, serving as a source of memories, images, and hopes when interpreted within a believing community. The second source was *tradition*, the residue of the corporate experience of earlier Christian communities. By tradition the Methodists meant both a specific historical and social horizon and a transcendent "environment of grace in and by which all Christians live, which is the continuation through time and space of God's self-giving love in Jesus Christ."

A third source for theological reflection was *experience*, understood as the appropriation of God's unmeasured mercy by persons and communities of persons who had been enabled to respond with trust and confidence.

And the fourth was *reason*, the continuing effort to avoid both self-contradiction and an unnecessary clash with the scientific and empirical wisdoms of the broader culture. The conference recognized that revelation and Christian experience could "transcend the scope of reason," yet they affirmed that all truth had its source in the God of truth, so that our efforts to discern the connections between faith and science, grace and nature, were useful endeavors in developing credible and communicable doctrine.[9]

The quadrilateral was a sensitive and accurate reflection of Wesley's own criteria of theological adequacy, and it had the additional merit of recognizing that traditions may change and develop without losing their coherence as traditions. The conference could both acknowledge and affirm the theological pluralism within the Methodist traditions, and yet it could also speak against the "theological indifferentism" that had been a part of Methodist history. It could acknowledge that the pluralism itself witnessed to the "transcendent mystery of divine truth" and yet insist that the marrow of Christian truth could be identified and conserved, even if it could not and ought not be stated in precisely defined propositions.[10]

Yet the theologians at that 1972 conference recognized that accepting four sources of theological reflection was only the beginning of the theological task. And our awareness of the quadrilateral is only the start of defining a Methodist tradition and mining its insights about health and healing. It is one thing to say that the four sources, in varying configurations, have indeed marked the Methodist tradition and have helped explain its continuing interest in health and healing. It is another to assume that by identifying formal criteria for reflection we have arrived at a satisfactory picture of a tradition.

For one thing, other traditions within the larger Christian tradition make a similar appeal to Scripture, tradition, experience, and reason. For another, the explication of formal criteria does not help us understand how the language and piety of the Methodist tradition have shaped a distinctive style of Christian existence and formed a Christian vision of health and healing, caring, and curing.

The task is not to propound a traditionalism that would bind the Methodist churches to any specific vision in their past. It would be foolish to argue that twentieth-century theologians must speak of sin and salvation in precisely the same language that Wesley used in the eighteenth century. It would be ludicrous to insist that because Wesley, in his *Primitive Physick*, disapproved the therapeutic use of Peruvian bark, the twentieth-century Methodist must entertain suspicions of quinine, which happened to be the chemical ingredient in the bark.

The more useful task is to understand how persons are formed by traditions and how some persons have been formed by this particular tradition. For we are shaped by traditions, whether we know it or not. We bear the mark of our broader past—a past that extends temporally beyond the boundaries of our isolated biographies—even when we are unable to recognize it or put it into words.

Three questions therefore guide our further reflection in this introductory chapter. What was the distinctive character of Wesley's own theological vision? How did he locate his views of health and medicine, curing and caring, within that broader vision? And how does that vision illumine for us the variety of ways in which we are formed and informed by traditions?

## SALVATION AND HEALTH IN THE CHRISTIAN JOURNEY

To talk about the distinctiveness of Wesley's theological vision is not simply to list the distinctive Wesleyan doctrines. Wesley did emphasize certain doctrines, and his contemporaries came to associate those doctrines with the Methodist movement, sometimes with disgust and sometimes with devotion. He wrote of prevenient grace, by which God invited and empowered every person to accept the gift of salvation; justification by faith, or God's forgiveness and pardon of all who accepted that gift; rebirth, the inward change that resulted from the new relation to God; and entire sanctification, the perfecting of the Christian in love. But this enumeration of doctrines fails to show how Wesley combined the pieces into a larger vision of the Christian life.

Wesley's metaphors often provide an illuminating guide to his theology. He returned continually, for example, to the image of "the way," to the challenge of persevering in the way and the dangers of being "turned out of the way" or of "mistaking the way." The image sometimes appeared in the titles of Wesley's better-known sermons: "The Scripture Way of Salvation," "The Way to the Kingdom," "The More Excellent Way." He spoke of the narrow path within the narrow way, or of higher and lower ways. Or, varying the image only slightly, Wesley could speak of the Christian's "walk." "To believe (in the Christian sense)," he once said, "is, then, to walk in the way of eternity."[11]

By "the way," Wesley meant the path of salvation. By salvation he meant not simply "a blessing which lies on the other side of death," in the "other world." It was not something at a distance. It was also not a momentary event, a punctiliar experience discontinuous with other experiences. With the term *salvation* Wesley wanted to designate the entire redemptive work of God, from the first dawning of grace in the soul to the final consummation. Salvation was a way of being in the world. It was a process of living and dying, again and again, often extending throughout a lifetime.[12]

The purpose of theology for Wesley was to mark the boundaries of that way, to provide guideposts that helped the Christian remain within the way. He eventually became convinced, moreover, that the center and substance of the way of salvation was love. He was unlike the sixteenth-century Protestant Reformers in his insistence that faith was subordinate to love, that faith was to be understood chiefly as a means for the restoration of love. Wesley could even say that faith lost all its excellence when brought into a comparison with love. Faith was merely the "handmaid" of love, for love was "the end, the sole end, of every dispensation of God, from the beginning of the world to the consummation of all things."[13]

The theologians at the 1972 United Methodist General Conference noted in their definition of "Our Theological Task" that "generally we have been more interested in relating doctrine to life than in speculative analysis. The ethical fruits of faith concern us more than systems of doctrine."[14] The statement acknowledged, on one level, that Methodists have often avoided the demands of conceptual clarity and definition. On another level, it affirmed a tradition that has taken ethical questions seriously, precisely in an effort to understand the limits and possibilities of the theme of love. It is no accident, then, that ethicists make frequent appearances in the pages of this volume.

Yet Wesley's references to faith as the handmaid of love surely must not be taken to mean that he conceived of the Christian life simply as a pattern of ethical behavior. However much Wesley's successors might have fallen into an unimaginative moralism that understood commitment to Christ simply as a matter of being good and doing good, Wesley himself always retained an intense awareness of the giftlike character of Christian existence.

His elevation of love did not, in his eyes, entail any diminution of faith. He was certain, after 1738, that love itself was impossible except as a fruit of faith. Wesley believed that faith was the sole condition of the Christian's being accepted and justified by God, and he agreed that faith was a gift of grace.

Faith for Wesley was something other than mere assent or belief. Faith was a conviction of things not seen, a conviction that God was in Christ reconciling the world. It was also a trust and confidence on the part of the Christian "that Christ died for my sins, that he loved me and gave himself for me." Or Wesley could speak of faith as the gift of seeing or hearing or tasting truths that would not have otherwise been seen or heard or tasted. From 1738 until the day he died, Wesley insisted that God's justification of the sinner issued solely from grace through faith.[15]

The Wesleyan style of theological reflection is rooted in Wesley's own struggle to maintain the proper ordering of faith and love. The task of theology, he thought, was to find the appropriate way between two erroneous extremes: on the one side, the error was a moralism that made love a means of salvation; on the other, an antinomianism that made faith an excuse for lovelessness.

Wesley liked the metaphor of journeying. When he was once accosted by a drunken and boorish traveler who barraged him with questions about his travels, Wesley responded, "Are you aware that we are on a longer journey; that we are traveling toward eternity?"[16] The metaphor of journeying helps us understand not only Wesley's own theological pilgrimage but also the final form in which he cast his thought.

Wesley was a priest of the Church of England, and he accepted the articles and liturgies which had emerged in that church following the Protestant Reformation of the sixteenth century. He stood within the "middle way" that Anglicanism tried to weave between Roman Catholicism and radical Protestantism. Hence Wesley thought of himself as an heir of the Reformation, but in the course of his spiritual odyssey he felt the formative influence of several Christian traditions.

During the early 1720s, Wesley felt entirely comfortable with the thought that by imposing a rigorous internal order on the affections he could build the loving life. Impressed by the Anglican theologians of "holy living"— especially Jeremy Taylor and William Law—he defined love as "purity of intention" and thought that by strict obedience to the law of love he could attain his salvation. But he found that a love flowing solely from internal discipline and order left him without confidence and trust. The way of moralism led to a dead end.

He slid, therefore, toward the other side of the way. During the late 1720s he experimented with what he later called a mystical quietism. He abandoned the ordered security of the law and began to seek the mystic union with God that brought freedom from excessive internal demands and from the command of God. "Love is all," he thought, and love is sheer spontaneity, issuing from an unreserved openness to God. "Thus were all the bands burst at once." But the bursting of the bands proved distracting. In the utter freedom of mystical faith, Wesley found himself "continually doubting whether I was right or wrong."[17]

During the early 1730s, therefore, he began to swing back once more.

While at Oxford he read deeply in the theologians of the early Church, especially Greek and Syrian writers, and began to reinterpret Christian holiness as a *disciplined* love. One could not, he concluded, force the loving disposition into existence; but one could also not assume that it simply sprang into being spontaneously within the faithful person. The loving life, he thought, would come gradually, as the Christian did works of charity and engaged in worship and devotion. If Wesley could adhere to the word and the sacraments, he thought, then he could find the way. But in fact he still found himself subject to despair. He was, he said, still "striving," rather than trusting.[18]

Wesley's struggle continued throughout his sojourn in America, where he felt the influence of yet another Christian tradition. On the way to Georgia he met a band of Moravians, the spiritual heirs of a fifteenth-century religious reformer named John Huss, whose early followers had designated themselves simply as the Unity of Brethren (*Unitas Fratrum*). The insistence of the Brethren on the sole authority of the Bible, the desirability of simplicity in worship, and the necessity of a disciplined life brought persecution and suffering, and it seemed at times that their churches would not survive.

In 1722, however, Brethren refugees from Moravia traveled to Count Nicholas von Zinzendorf's estate in Saxony. A German Lutheran, Zinzendorf had been profoundly affected by a reforming movement known as pietism, which in the seventeenth century brought to continental Protestants a new accent on inward experience, the practice of piety in small groups, service to the downtrodden, and missionary outreach. He introduced his Moravian friends to the spirituality of Lutheran pietism, and they adopted it as their own. Wesley's encounter with the Moravians in Georgia therefore added a new degree of richness and complexity to his own spiritual understanding.

On his return to England, Wesley met a Moravian missionary named Peter Boehler, who convinced him that the root of his dilemma was his misunderstanding of faith. Boehler told Wesley that he was still thinking of faith as simply hope and belief, not as trust and confidence. Faith, he said, was one's trust that one was forgiven. It was an insight that Wesley resisted, for if it were true, it meant that Wesley himself "had not faith." He disputed mightily with Boehler, trying to show that one could be faithful without having an assurance of being forgiven. But in his own judgment he lost the dispute, and that judgment was confirmed by his experience in the chapel on Aldersgate Street on May 24, 1738, when a reading of the preface to Luther's commentary on Romans served as the occasion for a new sense in Wesley that he did trust and that he felt assured.[19]

Yet the journey was by no means complete. In 1739 Wesley moved away from the Lutheran pietism that he had learned from the Moravians. They believed that faithfulness was all or nothing. They could not entertain the idea that there might be degrees of faith, that one could struggle still with doubt and fear and yet be faithful. Wesley disagreed: there could be degrees of faith. The Moravians believed, moreover, that the Christian without an assured faith should do nothing in order to obtain it. They called this their doctrine of stillness. One ought simply to wait, not to seek. Wesley disagreed: the word and sacraments were means of grace, and seeking Christians should use them. The Moravians believed, finally, that the Christian's only duty was to believe and to trust, not to perform good works. Christians might want to perform good works, they said, but they were not obliged to do so. Wesley disagreed: the law, the command to love, remained as a guide and a duty for even the faithful Christian.[20] So Wesley broke with the Moravians, and he began piecing together the elements of his theology to point the way between a legalistic love and a lawless faith.

Wesley believed that theologians drew maps for pilgrims, and because pilgrimages taxed the body as well as the soul, he had no hesitation about adding markers that could provide aid and comfort for the body. He never assumed that either the body or the mind stood outside the circle of theological concerns.

Because he organized his theological insights around the overarching image of a pilgrimage, Wesley spoke of sequences, stages, advances and lapses, forward movement. The Christian life was part of a vast movement from creation to consummation, and every Christian embodied, at the level of the microcosm, something of the larger movement of the cosmos itself. He maintained a pressing interest in what he called "the new creation," the coming transformation of all things, a change that would encompass not only the soul but the world. The new creation would be a change in the heavens and the earth, a change from disharmony to harmony and from ugliness to beauty. In the new creation, there would be no sickness, no pain, no death. Hence the struggle against sickness, pain, and death anticipated the larger end of creation, and that larger end continually informed each individual journey.[21]

Wesley's doctrine of creation had implications for every facet of his theology. For him the creation seemed to be a universal whole, without gaps or chasms, every part admirably connected to every other part. To express his vision of interconnectedness, Wesley appealed to the traditional notion of "one chain of beings, from the lowest to the highest point." An unbroken chain reached from the lowest element to the archangel Michael, from inorganic earth to human beings and angels. And the creation was good; indeed, it was "very good." Wesley believed that "the great Creator made nothing to be miserable, but every creature to be happy in its kind."[22]

Believing that the creation was good, Wesley viewed the natural sciences as forms of devotion. He thought that the clergy should be learned in "natural philosophy," and he himself read everything that he could find on the topic, including the works of Isaac Newton, the naturalist John Ray, and the popularizer William Derham. Wesley himself wrote occasionally on scientific matters, and he carried out simple experiments to enhance his understanding of electricity. He considered medicine a noble science not simply because of its therapeutic benefits but also because physicians discovered new secrets of nature.[23]

Wesley also insisted on the goodness of the body. It was, in his view, an "exquisitely wrought machine," and he was intensely curious about it and deeply respectful of its mysteries:

> What is flesh? That of the muscles in particular? Are the fibres that compose it of a determinate size? So that they can be divided only so far? Or are they resolvable *ad infinitum*? How does a muscle act? . . . Are the nerves pervious or solid? How do they act? By vibration or transmission of the animal spirits? Who knows what the animal spirits are? . . . What is sleep? Wherein does it consist? What is dreaming?[24]

The questions were important, Wesley thought, because we are the stewards of our bodies. God entrusted us with them, and we were to care for them as we would any precious gift.

The questions also were important, he thought, because our bodies help to constitute who we are. Wesley did not believe that the body served merely as a receptacle of the soul, or that the higher reaches of human thought were the act of a disembodied spirit. All the operations of the soul depended on bodily organs, especially on the brain. The soul and the body enjoyed a "natural union," with the result that thinking had to be understood as "the act of a spirit connected with a body and playing upon a set of material keys."[25]

Because he believed that the creation was good, finally, he assigned it a normative status in his narrative of salvation. The goal of redemption was none other than the restoration of the created harmony. Adam and Eve in the garden had been created in the "natural" image of God. They were creatures endowed with understanding, will, and liberty, and those capacities functioned in harmony with each other. They had also been created in the "political" image of God: they exercised wise and appropriate dominion over the remainder of the created order. And they had been created in the "moral" image of God: they shared the capacity for love. This depiction of creation provided a standard for what the human being could become. By God's grace, the original integrity could be restored. Salvation was a restoration of the created order, not a destruction of it. God's activity as redeemer did not overwhelm God's activity as creator. The aim of Christ's coming was to renew human nature in accordance with the pattern established in the creation.[26]

It was therefore of considerable importance to Wesley that the created order, in its integrity, included the proper ordering of the body. In the garden, Man and Woman needed no medication, for they knew no pain, sickness, weakness, or bodily disorder. The natural creation itself extended friendship to them: in paradise there was no injury. Hence the restoring of the created order through God's grace would also include the restoring of health to the physical body. Because creation was good, and because that goodness included health, then the healing of the body was in accord with the deepest nature of things. In Wesley's understanding of healing and health, the story of the garden functioned as a reminder that Christians were to take the physical flesh seriously.[27]

Yet Wesley knew that the present disorder, of the world and of the body, was not in accord with the deepest nature of things. Something had intervened, and Wesley believed, of course, that the intruder was sin. The doctrine of original sin was for him one of the fundamental convictions of Christian belief. Its proof was the universality of misery. When the enlightened clerics of his era called into question the old doctrine of original sin, Wesley accused them of sheer blindness. Everywhere he looked—to ancient Rome, to Africa and America, to China or Turkey, or to Italy, Germany, and England—Wesley found a history of cruelty, violence, stupidity, and greed.

His opponents attributed the disorder to the power of bad example, but why was "bad example" so prevalent throughout all known times and all known places? Wesley found the biblical doctrine of sinfulness much more convincing in its assertion that misery resulted from a flaw deeply ingrained in human nature, a flaw so terrible that it could be traced only to an absurd and arbitrary primal rebellion.[28]

Wesley did not assume that "original sin" or "total depravity" entailed an utter destruction of the image of God in the fallen creature. Rather than speaking of sin as an obliteration of the divine image, he preferred to describe it, in traditional Catholic terms, as a disease. But in using images of disease to describe the plight of the creature, Wesley did not intend to minimize the effects of sin. Every person, he thought, suffered from the disease of sinfulness, a disease with terrifying symptoms: pride, willfulness, self-deception, blindness, and a vast array of other disordered tempers. Indeed, he believed that to be infected with the disease of sinfulness was to be caught in the grip of a living death, a "spiritual death" that removed any possibility of happiness or health. And Wesley did not, after 1738, think that the living dead could heal themselves.[29]

They could not heal themselves because the seeds of sickness and death were lodged in their "inmost substance." As a consequence, sinfulness infected not only their souls but also their bodies. Being possessed by death, they discovered that the life-sustaining creation conspired against them. The sun and the moon shed unwholesome influence; the earth exhaled poisonous damps; the very air was "replete with the shafts of death." Even the food that they ate to sustain their lives sapped daily the very foundation of life. In that sense Wesley could speak of sickness and death as a punishment for sin. He was not saying that a child's illness was to be interpreted as a sign of God's vindictive wrath against the child, or that a premature death was to be construed as punishment for some specific sin. His contention, rather, was that the general human susceptibility to sickness and death could best be understood as a residue of the primal rebellion. In the fallen disorder, the forces of created order continually inflicted punishment on everyone.[30]

Sinfulness infected body and soul, and it also ensured that each would conspire against the other. Precisely because he could not accept a dualistic severing of the soul from the body in the original creation, Wesley had to assume that body and soul remained interdependent after the Fall. And since fallenness embraced both, he also had to assume that the corruptible body could destroy the soul and the corruptible soul destroy the body.

The body, drained by infirmities, subverted the capacities of the soul, or spirit. Wesley had no difficulty whatsoever with the suggestion that defects of the spirit—defects of judgment or imagination—could flow "from the natural constitution of the body." A diseased brain could produce delirium of spirit, disordered nerves could engender distempered thoughts, and obstructed circulation could create spiritual temptations.

> Consider, first, the nature of the body with which your soul is connected. How many are the evils which it is every day, every hour, liable to. Weakness, sickness, and disorders of a thousand kinds, are its natural attendants. Consider the inconceivably minute fibres, threads, abundantly finer than hair, (called from thence capillary vessels,) whereof every part of it is composed; consider the innumerable multitude of equally fine pipes and strainers, all filled with circulating juice. And will not the

breach of a few of these fibres, or the obstruction of a few of these tubes, particularly in the brain, or heart, or lungs, destroy our ease, health, strength, if not life itself? Now if we observe that all pain implies temptation, how numberless must the temptations be, which will beset every man, more or less, sooner or later, while he dwells in this corruptible body![31]

Wesley would not have shied away from the assertion that spiritual despair might well be simply a reflection of chemical imbalance.

He was not saying that the body was itself sinful. He thought it absurd to talk about a "sinful body." Spirits alone, he said, are capable of sin. But spirits lived as bodies. They did not simply live in bodies; they remained "in vital union" with bodies. The spirit could not "exert any of its operations, any otherwise than in union with the body, with its bodily organs." So if sinfulness disordered the body, the spirit, too, would suffer.[32]

By the same token, the spirit, drained by infirmities, subverted the capacities of the body. Wesley was impressed by the tendency of spiritual malaise to find bodily expression. The disordered passions, he thought, had a far "greater influence on health than most people are aware of." Violent and sudden passions were likely to "dispose to, or actually throw people into acute diseases." Slow and enduring passions, like grief and hopeless love, were likely to "bring on chronical diseases." Until the passion was calmed, medicine was applied in vain. And as long as the disorder of sinfulness confused the soul, the passion would remain uncalmed.[33]

Because of this vision of sinfulness, therefore, Wesley described our living as a living-toward-death. And he depicted that state in graphic detail: human bodies, he said, began their existence filled with innumerable membranes, exquisitely thin, in which fluids continually circulated. But when they aged, the bodies stiffened; the arteries themselves, the grand instruments of circulation, became stiff and hard, unable to propel the blood through even the largest channels. And the result was death. "Thus are the very seeds of death sown in our very nature. Thus from the very hour when we first appear on the stage of life, we are traveling towards death: we are preparing, whether we will or no, to return to the dust from whence we came."[34]

Wesley's sensitivity to the subtleties of what we call psychosomatic illness reflected a Christian doctrine of creation and fall. His doctrine of creation manifested his convictions about the integrity of the created order, which entailed for him the integral unity of body and soul. His doctrine of the Fall exhibited his convictions about the disintegration of the created order, which entailed that both the body and the soul fell into disharmony. But the Fall did not sever the body from the soul, and it was therefore clear that salvation must somehow encompass the whole person—body and soul in unity.

Salvation for Wesley was "a restoration of the soul to its primitive health." He spoke of it mainly with therapeutic metaphors. Religion, in its proper nature, was the "therapy of the soul."[35] "It is *therapeia psyches*, God's method of healing a soul which is . . . diseased. Hereby the great Physician of souls applies medicines to heal this sickness; to restore human nature, totally corrupted in all its faculties."[36] The healing encompassed such spiritual diseases as pride and self-will, but the grand purpose was to restore not simply the soul but the entirety of the "human nature," including the body. For such an audacious project, the Physician's prescription was simple and yet demanding: the soul had to embark on a journey.

Every step of the way was a fruit of "free grace." The "natural free will" lacked the capacity even to begin the trip. Only the soul empowered by the gift of grace could set out on the journey, and the gift that began the journey was God's "prevenient grace"—a light that glimmered in every soul.[37] Like a number of other Anglican theologians, Wesley believed that no man or woman was entirely destitute of grace. The only persons who existed in a state of "mere nature" were those who had willfully and persistently resisted the gracious promptings of the Spirit, and they were few. Most men and women had at least the capacity to recognize their sinful nature. What was commonly called "natural conscience" seemed to Wesley a gracious gift through which God awakened in the sinful soul the first "slight transient conviction of having sinned." That conviction implied some "tendency towards life," some slight degree of salvation, the beginning of deliverance.[38]

For men and women at the outset of the journey, physical illness might well serve as an occasion for the conscience to recognize the perilous state of the soul. Illness, Wesley thought, had a way of humbling the prideful. And though the illness itself was no gracious gift, the self-recognition that it sometimes evoked could bear within it the beginnings of a new and better future. In any case, Wesley would have thought that the self-recognition was no achievement in which to take pride, for he did not consider self-awareness to be a consequence of calculation. It was, rather, a gift.

For the awakened, the journey proceeded by means of God's "convincing grace," which the Scripture usually designated as "repentance." The initial recognition of one's sinfulness implied a sense of regret, and that first "slight transient conviction" could shade gradually into a deeper sorrow. Wesley never tried to define precisely the point at which conviction became repentance; he argued, rather, that the transition was a matter of degree. Repentance was "a larger measure of self-knowledge," and like the awareness by which it was elicited, repentance, too, was a gift, not an achievement.[39]

In giving the gift, however, God the Giver retained always an invariable respect for the recipient's integrity. Wesley insisted that God saved men and women "as reasonable creatures, endued with understanding to discern what is good, and liberty either to accept or refuse it." God did not treat sinners as stones; God did not coerce the will. Wesley preferred to speak of God as drawing or wooing the soul, which, because of the gift of prevenient grace, could respond with faith and love to the Giver.[40]

Repentance served as the prelude to faith, and Wesley believed, with the Protestant Reformers, that through grace the sinful soul was saved by faith. Faith alone permitted the soul to drop its defenses; faith alone permitted the sinful self to trust "that God is reconciled to me through his Son." Wesley preached consistently after 1738 the message of justification by grace through faith. By justification, he said, we are saved from the guilt of sin and restored to the favor of God. And justification for Wesley was more than just a pronouncement of forgiveness; it was also a healing, restorative act. It was the beginning of a convalescence, the beginning of faith's own journey.[41]

So remarkable was the transition from faithlessness to faith that Wesley could describe it only as a "rebirth," analogous to the birth of a child who in the womb had been unable to see or to hear. Even that analogy failed to capture the full mystery of rebirth, for a child in the womb was alive even before birth, while the sinful soul was spiritually dead before God granted it life. Hence justification for Wesley necessarily had its subjective correlate in rebirth.

> If any doctrines within the whole compass of Christianity may be properly termed fundamental, they are doubtless these two: the doctrine of justification, and that of the new birth: the former relating to that great work which God does *for* us; the latter, to the great work which God does *in* us, in renewing our fallen nature.[42]

Though the two events—justification and rebirth—were simultaneous, the rebirth, he thought, had to be considered as the fruit of the justification. And the rebirth began a new stage in the soul's journey.

Yet the further journey was more than a pilgrimage of the soul, for the soul was embodied. Just as Wesley affirmed the interdependence of soul and body, so also he affirmed the interconnection of salvation and health.

Just as he saw sickness and death as consequences of the Fall, so also he saw healing and life as fruits of salvation.

In making those connections, Wesley was taking a dangerous path. He ran the risk of seeming to imply that the truly faithful Christian should somehow transcend the ills of body and mind. He ran the additional risk of seeming to suggest a utilitarian conception of faithfulness as merely a means to a human end, worship as a means of health. Certainly he did not intend to make such a suggestion, but the risk was real.

His understanding of salvation, though, required that he run that risk. He did not conceive of salvation simply as a future life in another world; it was the "entire work of God in the soul," from the first dawnings of spiritual life to the final consummation. For Wesley the term *salvation* referred to a process that could continue throughout a lifetime. It was a way of being in the world. Therefore his notion of salvation inevitably raised questions about the relationship between salvation and health. Could one say, for instance, that a person trapped within the agony of mental illness, a person utterly distraught and despondent as a result of, say, chemical imbalance in the brain, might yet partake meaningfully of the gift of salvation?

Wesley assumed, after all, that salvation brought not only holiness but also happiness. Like Augustine and Thomas Aquinas, he believed that human beings were naturally oriented to happiness. True religion produced holiness and happiness; the kingdom of God was holiness and happiness. In making such assertions, Wesley was by no means departing from the consensus of eighteenth-century English Christians. It had long been a theological commonplace that human activity reflected a natural desire for happiness, and that salvation was the fulfillment of happiness, not its negation. Because he conceived of salvation as an extended process in this life, Wesley faced the question of the relations among holiness, happiness, and health. Did it not seem that meaningful participation in the life of salvation required at least a bare minimum of what we would call mental health?[43]

Wesley implicitly dealt with that question in his descriptions of the later stages of salvation. He believed that rebirth initiated a process of "sanctification," a process through which the Christian was gradually restored to the image of God. Justification offered salvation from the guilt of sin and restoration to God's favor; sanctification provided salvation from the power of sin and restoration of God's image. "It begins," Wesley said, "the moment we are justified, in the holy, humble, gentle, patient love of God and man." And it gradually increased from that moment, just as a grain of mustard seed gradually became a great tree.[44]

The heart of sanctification was the capacity to love. When Wesley talked about the Christian's growth, he meant the enhancement of the capacity to love. Holiness was the faithful and joyous love of God and neighbor, nothing less. Neither eloquence nor knowledge, neither faith nor works, neither rejoicing nor suffering could avail without love. The bedrock of the gospel was "a peaceful, joyous love of God" and a patient and gentle love of the neighbor.[45]

Had Wesley said no more, his doctrine of sanctification would have evoked little dissent from his contemporaries. But we went on to say that gradual sanctification could, through God's grace, issue in a capacity for "perfect love," even in this life. In an instant, a moment within the longer process, the Christian could receive the gift—and Wesley never doubted that it was a gift—of "pure love" for God and neighbor.[46]

So Wesley could talk of Christian perfection, meaning the perfection of love. His doctrine evoked scorn and suspicion, but he refused to yield. He disliked the phrase "sinless perfection," but he believed that love could become the "sole principle of action" for a man or woman, and, in that narrow sense, that the Christian could "live without sin." The doctrine sounded—and sounds—audacious.[47]

Under the pressure of criticism, he tried to define his position with care. Wesley acknowledged that even the Christian who had received the gift of perfect love—the gift of "entire sanctification"—could be liable to mistakes in judgment, which could occasion "transgression of the perfect law." But he thought that the transgression was not properly "sinful" if it proceeded from a consistent temper of love. Christians could never be so perfect as to be free from ignorance and mistakes. But they could refrain from voluntary outward sins, and they could be free of evil thoughts and tempers, and they could love God with all their heart, mind, soul, and strength.[48]

Christian perfection was not a state marking the end of the Christian journey. When Wesley used the term *perfection*, he meant a "perfecting" that lured the pilgrim onward. He refused to speak of "absolute perfection." He thought that there was no perfection "which does not admit of a continual increase." Perfection was a way, not a static goal. And the Christians who walked the way of perfect love remained within the common pilgrimage. They, too, shared the common need to grow in grace, "daily to advance in the knowledge and love of God."[49]

Wesley felt certain that the way of love brought healing to the soul. He also thought that it could bring health to the mind and body. Because the soul was embodied, its dispositions altered the body through which it lived. Wesley once encountered a woman who had continual pain in her stomach.

Her physicians had prescribed drug upon drug, without effect. Their mistake, he thought, was that they ignored the root of her disorder:

> Whence came this woman's pain? (which she would never have told, had she never been questioned about it:) from fretting for the death of her son. And what availed medicines, while this fretting continued? Why then do not all physicians consider how far bodily disorders are caused or influenced by the mind; and in those cases, which are utterly out of their sphere, call in the assistance of a minister; as ministers, when they find the mind disordered by the body, call in the assistance of a physician?[50]

The woman suffered from physical maladies, he thought, because her grief had overwhelmed her capacity for joyous love.

Wesley was aware, as many have been aware, that tranquility of the spirit could be physically therapeutic.

> The love of God, as it is the sovereign remedy of all miseries, so in particular it effectually prevents all the bodily disorders the passions introduce, by keeping the passions themselves within due bounds. And by the unspeakable joy and perfect calm, serenity and tranquility it gives the mind, it becomes the most powerful of all the means of health and long life.[51]

He could therefore speak of love as the "medicine" of life, the "never-failing remedy" for the evils of a disordered world, and all the miseries and vices of men and women.[52]

Lest anyone assume, however, that love was merely a means to improved health, Wesley also emphasized that even the soul perfected by love often had to endure the ills of the "shattered body." The disorder of the body, in fact, could limit the disposition of love. Inner disorder—the proneness to disease—led to confused apprehensions, false judgments, wrong inferences, and grievous mistakes, even in mature Christians, and such maladies, while they could not destroy the loving temper, could hinder it. Sickness could engender a humility that was receptive to the gift of love, but sickness could also engender lovelessness.[53]

By implication, therefore, Wesley proposed an answer to the question about salvation and health. He suggested that the utter absence of health probably would, in some instances at least, preclude any meaningful participation in the process of salvation. Wesley talked of degrees of salvation, and he believed that the higher levels of salvation clearly presupposed a capacity for love. To the degree that severe mental or physical distress hindered that capacity for love, it hindered a full participation in the perfecting of love. Wesley never assumed, of course, that even the most crippling ill-ness could finally overcome God's invincible love, but for him the chief proof of that invincibility was the likelihood that God would open new possibilities in another life beyond this one. Yet Wesley understood salva-tion as being far more than "a life beyond this one," and the Wesleyan understanding of salvation as a process implied that the Christian who truly cared about salvation might also have to care about health.

On one level, then, Wesley's interest in health and medicine reflected his concerns about the salvation of souls. When he instructed his "visitors" about the proper care for the sick, he told them to inquire about the needs of both body and spirit. But he never suggested that they should consider the health of the spirit merely as a means to the health of the body. His con-stant assumption was that they cared for the body because they cared for the salvation of the person. His understanding of care for the sick embraced, in fact, a pastoral strategy, namely, that it might be necessary for the Christian pastor, lay or ordained, to address the issue of health as the pre-lude to addressing the larger issue of salvation.[54]

On another level, Wesley's interest in health and medicine reflected his sense of the duties implicit in love. Caring for the sick, he said, helped to form and discipline love. In that sense, care for the sick became a means of grace to the visitor who cared. But to care for the sick was also to express love, and in that sense caring became a way simply of living the life of love.

One finds it difficult to disentangle Wesley's manifold labors on behalf of the sick from his theological sensitivity to the theme of love. He would not himself have described that sensitivity as merely ethical, though surely it helps to explain the ethical preoccupations of the Wesleyan tradition. For Wesley, the notion of love was deeply embedded within the self-understanding of a community that was formed by its common journey. And in that journey, Christians cared for the sick because it was the loving thing to do.[55]

## THE USES OF TRADITION

Images of journeying have reappeared frequently throughout the devel-opment of the Methodist tradition. In fact, one can understand some of the critical divisions within the tradition as reflections of disagreements about the proper progression within the order of salvation. "Holiness" churches emerged in the nineteenth century in the wake of charges that mainline Methodists had become satisfied with the "first blessing" of pardon and forgiveness and insufficiently concerned about moving onward to the "second blessing" of holiness. Pentecostal churches emerged in the wake of similar charges that the holiness groups had lingered at the "second blessing" and failed to press on toward the "third blessing" of charismatic ecstasy.

Within the mainline Methodist traditions, the notion of Christian existence as a journey has persisted. The General Conference of the United Methodists spoke for the larger Methodist family in 1972 when it described the Methodist churches as a "pilgrim people under the Lordship of Christ." Methodist theologians have long retained an understanding of theology as a practical discipline, and most of them would agree that the function of theology is to guide and inform a pilgrim people.[56]

Methodists interested in obtaining guidance about health and medicine have appealed to their tradition in diverse ways. The first and most obvious way has simply been a straightforward appeal to precedent. When Methodists in America wished to create support for the building of hospitals in the early twentieth century, they reminded the denomination that "the founder of Methodism, like his Master, went everywhere preaching and teaching and healing the sick; and he studied medicine that he might heal the bodies of men while ministering to their spiritual needs." They found in Wesley's example of "systematically and scientifically caring for the sick poor" a persuasive motive for Methodists to resume the task of medical service.[57]

A second use of tradition appeared in the organization during the nineteenth century of a deaconess movement which assumed as one of its responsibilities the care of the sick. Eighteenth-century Methodists had not created a formal organization of deaconesses, but certain features of the early Methodist movement help to explain the later appearance of such organizations.

Not only had women made up a majority of the eighteenth-century Methodists but also they had assumed positions of leadership. Women occasionally led the Methodist "classes," the small groups at the heart of the movement. They exhorted and expounded texts within the class meetings, and although the early Methodists did not formally accept women as preachers, a few like Sarah Crosby and Mary Bosanquet Fletcher did, in fact, preach, even traveling through the countryside in the manner of the regular itinerant preachers. Observing that "Phoebe the deaconess" (Romans 16:1–2) had been "a visitor of the sick," Wesley encouraged women to become official visitors within the Methodist societies, charging them with the duty of seeing every sick person in their district three times a week. Thus was established a custom of asking women to care for the sick.[58]

The custom created no enduring institutional structures until the last quarter of the nineteenth century, when German and Swiss Methodists founded the Methodist deaconess movement, which began its work by training young women to serve as nurses in hospitals and homes. The movement eventually spread to Austria, Russia, Yugoslavia, Hungary, and the United States. Annie Wittenmeyer, an Ohio Methodist who had worked with the wounded during the Civil War, made a trip to Germany to observe the work of the deaconesses. Returning to America, where she had already organized a vast project in visitation by pious Methodist women, Wittenmeyer helped to popularize the notion of a deaconess corps.

The idea took root, and in 1885 Lucy Rider Meyer, a former chemistry professor who had attended the Woman's Medical College of Philadelphia to prepare herself as the wife of a medical missionary, opened a training school in Chicago which included studies in "hygiene, in citizenship, in social and family relationships, in everything that could help or hinder in the establishment of the Kingdom of Heaven on earth." The idea spread rapidly to other cities.[59]

Firmly established in 1888, the deaconess movement represented an early expression of the social gospel, sponsoring not only care for the sick but also other ministries within urban slums. Meyer eventually gained a medical degree from Northwestern University; the courses at her training school ranged from medicine to biblical studies, from church history to singing. Eventually the practice of caring for the sick in a few rooms of the school led to the creation of a hospital. And she soon had imitators: the New England Deaconess Home and Training School, founded in 1889, offered one course of study for nurses and another for other religious vocations, but it continued her vision of medical training as an expression of a social gospel.[60]

By the end of the century, more than six hundred Methodist women toiled as deaconesses in America, Germany, and Switzerland, caring for the sick in homes and hospitals and visiting the poor and unchurched in their tenements and hovels. The patterns of activity and expectation that were established in the eighteenth century thereby endured into the nineteenth and thus helped prepare the way for the deaconesses, their hospitals, and their social ministries.[61]

A third use of a tradition is to recover and interpret its ideas, and a few Methodist theologians have attempted an informed assessment of modern theories and techniques of health and healing by evaluating them in the light of the tradition's central theological affirmations. The American theologian Albert Outler, for example, has drawn on Wesleyan themes in examining the practice of psychotherapy. Outler's *Psychotherapy and the*

*Christian Message* (1954) sought areas of agreement between theology and psychology, but he also emphasized the need for theology to restrain the uncritical pretensions of a secularist psychotherapy.

Outler believed that exposure to the theories of psychotherapy had improved pastoral practice. It had encouraged self-awareness, checked clerical moralism, demonstrated the hidden and distorted sources of much religious thought and feeling, compelled a greater sense of respect for troubled and troublesome people, and clarified an understanding of human growth. He did not want the churches to lose sight of the "practical wisdom" of psychotherapy.

He was convinced, however, that the Christian world view provided a perspective for psychotherapy more adequate than any secularist faith could offer. Christian theologians, he said, recognized that our consciousness of ourselves as natural beings manifested our capacity to transcend nature and therefore to exercise some degree of "responsible freedom." They understood, moreover, that the discrepancy between the human quandary and human possibility resulted from a refusal to accept finitude, and hence from an unfaith and mistrust deeper than any specific neurotic maladjustment. They saw that self-fulfillment presupposed "a power at work in life and history . . . which moves in us and draws us into its mysterious workings." And finally, they grasped the paradoxical truth that self-fulfillment required self-denial (specifically, the "denial of self-importance") as its invariable condition.[62]

Outler devoted much of his career to the study of Wesley, and it is hardly surprising that the theological motifs he found most useful in his exploration of psychotherapy—human freedom, the human flaw, human possibility, forgiveness, and love—happened also to be the themes that he accented in his studies of Wesley. In Outler's work the interpretation of the tradition provided the categories for evaluating a therapeutic practice.

It is possible, finally, to argue for a fourth way in which the Methodist tradition has served as a resource for theological reflection on medical issues: it has formed attitudes and dispositions which find expression in patterns of argument and judgment. A religious tradition is far more than a set of doctrines, and Methodists, especially, have been formed religiously not so much by the catechism as by the hymnal. Methodism took shape in the eighteenth-century revivals, and it has always borne a residue of the revivalist's call for inwardness, for heart-felt experience, for decision, and for ethical fidelity.

To inquire into a Methodist tradition is to discover almost invariably the assumption that the church is not so much the repository of doctrinal truth as it is the community within which persons are formed. The heart of the tradition lies in hymns and prayers, corporate confession and moments of meditation, readings from the Old Testament and from the New, repeated week after week, year after year. Of course it is impossible to demonstrate that nurture within such a tradition can shape specific judgments about difficult issues in health and medicine. Yet it seems plausible, at least to a Methodist, that a lifetime, or even a childhood, spent within such a tradition can form a distinctive way of looking at things.

The American theologian Paul Ramsey once had occasion to reflect on his experience of growing up as a member of a small, conservative Methodist church in the Deep South and its possible imprint on his later thought. Ramsey has written extensively about medicine and health, on topics ranging from conception to death and dying, from abortion to the giving of vital organs, from in vitro fertilization to heart transplants. He also happens to be a Methodist layman, and one finds in his work a number of traditional Wesleyan motifs: the theme of love, the notion of righteousness, a concern for personal morality as well as for social justice, a high evaluation of the insights to be derived from the wisdom of the larger Christian tradition, a defense of the place of rules in Christian ethics, and a sense of our common existence as "a covenant people on a common pilgrimage."[63]

When Ramsey reflected on his years of nurture in a Methodist congregation, he found that his later ethical and theological judgments seemed strikingly congruent with some of his formative experiences. He recalled hearing his father, John Ramsey, the minister of the congregation, read each year in all his churches Wesley's rules for his societies, the rules about "fleeing the wrath to come, and going on to perfection, by doing all good, and avoiding every evil." And he speculated that his approach to the issues of medical ethics might well reflect, at some elusive level, "a deeply entrenched feeling and judgment [within the Methodist tradition which formed his early religious life] that there are some things a Christian should *never* do."[64]

Ramsey's reminiscences were filled with the words *maybe* and *possibly*, as indeed they would have to be. Who of us can isolate with certainty the sources in our past that formed our particular way of understanding the world, our characteristic style of argument, or our vision of the Christian faith? The sources are manifold and overlapping, complex beyond recovery, hidden largely from ourselves as well as from the psychoanalysts and sociologists and historians who try to explain human behavior. Yet we begin to understand the power of a tradition only when we glimpse the ways in which it forms attitudes, dispositions, and propensities which find expression in conceptual judgments but which could never be reduced to a list of propositions transmitted from one generation to another.

Some Methodists, then, have found in their tradition a source of precedents which have guided their participation in one or another specific project; others have reflected in their characteristic activities some enduring feature of Methodist institutional history; still others have found in the Wesleyan past a source of theological insight; and many others have borne, often unwittingly, the dispositional residues of their formation within local Methodist congregations. A study of health and medicine in the Wesleyan tradition must therefore embody something of the complexity within the tradition, as well as the variety of ways in which the tradition has shaped its sons and daughters.

It is appropriate that such a study assume a narrative shape, that it be a history recounting a movement rather than a systematic arrangement of designated topics. It will reveal not so much a set of fixed conclusions as a style of religious reflection, conducted often by Christians who disagree with each other about matters large and small. It will be a story not of people who have arrived, but of people who are on the way, whether to perfection or to an unknown future. It will be a story of a people undertaking a journey.

# ·2·

# Healing and Health

Wesley once visited an eminently pious woman who had been confined to her bed for several months, unable to raise herself up. At her request, he prayed that she might be healed of her malady. The result, as Wesley reported it, was that she rose, dressed herself, came downstairs, and had no further complaints. But Wesley also once visited a friend whom he found suffering with the symptoms of pleurisy. On hearing of the friend's distress, Wesley advised that he apply a brimstone plaster. The result, as Wesley reported it, was that in a few hours the friend was perfectly well. A multitude of similar experiences of both kinds soon convinced him that "God has more than one method of healing either the soul or the body." Healing, in Wesley's view, could be either natural or supernatural, and it could occur through both medication and prayer.[1]

In every instance, Wesley considered prayer to be an appropriate response to illness. In some, he thought, God responded immediately to the prayer in a miracle of healing. In others, God healed the body through the "natural" means of medication or surgery. He thought that the sick had every right to appeal for a miraculous healing, but that they also should have the prudence to use medicines wisely. He often prayed with them, but he also prescribed medicines for them.

The Methodist tradition has maintained both a sense of the appropriateness of prayer and a trust in the wisdom of medical science. But it has not done so without a struggle. Wesley's practice of praying for the sick suggested to some of his successors in the nineteenth century that spiritual healing—accomplished solely through prayer and faith—stood near the heart of the Wesleyan heritage. But other Methodists viewed efforts at spiritual healing as presumptuous superstition. The ensuing controversy created a division within the tradition that has never fully disappeared.

An understanding of Methodist conceptions of health and healing requires some grasp of old divisions within the tradition. Those divisions become understandable against the backdrop of Wesley's own activities as a healer of the body. He held in balance two conceptions of sickness and healing, which he designated as the "natural" and the "preternatural," or "supernatural," which lay beyond the boundaries of the natural order. In the course of the nineteenth century, the balance collapsed.[2]

Underlying the collapse were two conflicting visions of the Christian journey. The advocates of spiritual healing tended to think of Christian holiness as the result of a distinctive, specifiable experience, a moment of discontinuity that elevated the soul to a higher dimension of spiritual life. Conceiving of the holy life as the consequence of a supernatural crisis that produced a victory over sinfulness, they had no difficulty envisioning other supernatural interventions that could produce similar victories over sickness.

The advocates of medical healing tended to think of holiness as a gradual movement toward spiritual maturity, a process that formed human character and expanded its capacity for openness to God and other persons. Conceiving of the holy life as a gradual process through which the natural capacities were formed and reformed, they preferred to think of healing as a process that occurred in and through God's activities within the natural order. Both groups maintained a considerable interest in health and healing. Both could appeal to Wesley in support of their views.

## WESLEY AS HEALER

Wesley was no bustling example of good health. Almost certainly his interest in medicine resulted partly from his own struggle to overcome a constant array of bodily ills. To read Wesley's journals is to discover a distressing sequence of fevers, fits, nosebleeds, coughs, and consumption. When he was about twenty-seven, he began for several years to spit blood. He almost died from a fever. He suffered for a period from consumption. His hands often shook. He claimed when he was sixty-eight that he was then far healthier than he had been forty years earlier, but he soon had to undergo minor surgery for a swelling of the testicle.[3]

For whatever reasons, he began as a student of seventeen at Christ Church, Oxford, to read books on "anatomy and physic," and he continued to study those topics the rest of his life. His ambition to serve as a missionary in Georgia renewed his interest in medicine, for he thought that he might "be of some service to those who had no regular physician among them," and he continued his private medical studies after arriving in America. But it was not until 1746, long after he had returned to England, that Wesley made healing an integral part of his Methodist revival.[4]

When he began his healing venture in 1746, he meant by *healing* the practice of medicine. Moved by the spectacle of widespread illness and suffering among the poor, Wesley looked initially to the existing English hospitals as a source of relief. The hospitals offered little help. He sought the advice of licensed physicians. They offered little help. So as a "desperate expedient," Wesley decided that he himself would practice medicine. He again resumed his medical studies, aided this time by an apothecary and an experienced surgeon, and soon opened dispensaries in London, Bristol, and Newcastle, where he met patients for diagnosis and treatment.[5]

He spent each Friday seeing the sick, who came to him in large numbers. When his first patient told him that he had suffered from a cough for sixty years, Wesley feared that his inevitable failure to cure him would discourage others from coming, but Wesley's prescription seemed to help the man, and in the first five months, he dispensed medicines to about five hundred patients. He claimed that at least seventy-one of them were cured of distempers that had been thought incurable. Thereafter he occasionally recorded in his journal the number of patients who came each year, the number who took the medications and submitted to a proper regimen, and the number who were thereby cured of "diseases they had long laboured under."[6]

Resolved not to go beyond his depth, he dealt only with chronic illnesses, not with acute ones. He referred the difficult cases to licensed physicians. But his modesty did not preclude criticism from eighteenth-century doctors and twentieth-century historians, who often viewed him as an impertinent quack. Some of his prescriptions certainly sounded dubious: Wesley trusted the healing qualities of tar-water and sea-water, radish juice and garlic, and marigold flowers and Spanish snuff.[7]

His remedies hardly seemed ludicrous, though, in an era when physicians regularly prescribed bleeding and purges, opium and quicksilver, and blisters and plasters, or else placed *their* trust in the healing qualities of tar-water and sea-water, radish juice and garlic, or marigold flowers and Spanish snuff. In his own context, most of Wesley's prescriptions were mild. Medicine was hardly an advanced scientific enterprise. The medical curriculum was highly theoretical and speculative, and in any case Oxford graduated only about four physicians a year, Cambridge only a few more. Consequently, medical practice rested largely in the hands of apothecaries, who saw the patients and either issued prescriptions themselves or sought advice from physicians who rarely saw the patients. Wesley knew little about medicine, but neither did the physicians.[8]

In most medical matters, Wesley remained keenly aware that his knowledge had severe limits. About the therapeutic capacities of electricity, though, his enthusiasm knew few bounds. He observed experiments with electricity as early as 1747, and by 1753 he was testing its curative powers. He soon decided that it was "far superior to all the other medicines I have known. . . . Certainly it comes the nearest to an universal medicine of any yet known in the world." Electricity, for Wesley, was "a thousand medicines in one," and he thought it "the most efficacious medicine, in nervous disorders of every kind, which has ever yet been discovered." In 1756 he secured an electrical apparatus to treat anyone willing to try "the virtue of this surprising medicine," and before long he was electrifying patients throughout London.[9]

Wesley questioned the "sense" and "honesty" of physicians who scoffed at the use of electricity or questioned its safety. He believed that "hundreds, perhaps thousands" had received "unspeakable good" from the electrical devices, and he knew of no man, woman, or child who had "received any hurt thereby." He kept abreast of the literature on electricity, reading the reports of such scientists as Benjamin Franklin and Joseph Priestly, and in 1759 he published a compilation of the latest writings in his *Desideratum: or, Electricity made Plain and Useful.* In the introduction he admitted that electricity was no panacea, but he hastened to say that it was the "closest thing" to one, and he urged men and women of good sense to go ahead and use it, confident that it would prevent sickness and pain and save lives.[10]

His enthusiasm outran his judgment. Medical science later discovered beneficial therapeutic properties in the use of electricity, but Wesley admitted that nobody in the eighteenth century understood the theory of electricity, and he carried out his medical experiments in the face of criticism from both Priestly and Franklin, as well as from most physicians. The dosages were so small that they could hardly have caused harm, and Wesley himself underwent frequent treatment along with the other enthusiastic patients. But Wesley was experimenting with a medium that he did not understand, and he made claims on its behalf that he should not have made.

Yet the therapeutic use of electricity did illustrate Wesley's commitment to a scientific medicine that would be in harmony with knowledge of the natural world. Wesley certainly did not consider electricity to be a supernatural force accessible only to the faithful. He thought of it as an active force diffused throughout space, and he considered its therapeutic use to be the result of increased knowledge of nature. His own use of it exemplified his trust in the healing properties of natural forces.[11]

Wesley's interest in the work of physicians led him to edit for publication some of their popular writings. In 1769 he published his *Advice With Respect to Health*, a set of extracts from the Swiss physician Dr. Simon A. D. Tissot, whose views were compatible with Wesley's preferences for physical exercise, cheap and simple medicines, and outward applications rather than internal medications. In 1774 he published *An Extract from Dr. Cadogan's Dissertation on the Gout, and all Chronic Diseases*, a compilation of writings by William Cadogan, who also shared Wesley's enthusiasm for exercise and moderation in food and drink. One of Wesley's few criticisms of Cadogan's book was for its condemnation of wines, which Wesley considered "some of the most powerful medicines yet known." But he liked the book's warnings against intemperance, indolence, and excessive passions of either anger or joy.[12]

Wesley went beyond merely editing the work of others. In 1745 he published his first medical tract, *A Collection of Receipts for the Use of the Poor*, recommending simple cures for 63 illnesses. In 1747 he released his *Primitive Physick: An Easy and Natural Way of Curing Most Diseases*, containing remedies for about 250 maladies of every variety. Wesley took great pride in the book, thought it a great pity that any Methodist should be without it, and urged his preachers to distribute it along with his devotional treatises: "If you love the souls or bodies of men," he told one of them, "recommend, everywhere, the 'Primitive Physic' and the small tracts."[13]

The preachers must have loved souls and bodies, for the book went through twenty-three editions during Wesley's lifetime, and publishers continued to issue it long after his death. In substance, it was no great innovative tract. Wesley drew heavily, though selectively, on the work of such physicians as George Cheyne and "the great and good Dr. [Thomas] Sydenham." His rules for health in the book were taken mainly from Cheyne's *Book of Health and Long Life*. But what it lacked in wit or originality it made up for in its accessibility to the "plain" and the "poor," for it was Wesley's intention to teach every person with common sense to prescribe medications that would do no harm even when they could do no good. He wanted to provide "cheap, safe, and easy medicines" that could be applied by "plain, unlettered" men and women. And the plain people made his book the eighteenth-century equivalent of a best seller.[14]

Despite its practical intent, the book also represented Wesley's interest in one of the eighteenth century's spirited medical debates. The medical theorists who occupied the university chairs believed that medicine could become a science only when its practitioners achieved clarity about fundamental principles, which would become axioms that enabled one to deduce practical rules for therapy. Hence they considered medicine to be "an abstruse science, quite out of the reach of ordinary men." And they labeled the ragtag apothecaries as mere "empiricks," who worked by trial and error and healed only by accident.[15]

The empirics had their learned defenders, and Wesley joined forces with them: "And has not the author of nature taught us the use of many other medicines," he asked, "by what is vulgarly term'd accident?" The virtue of the empirics, he thought, was that their everyday experiences exploded the hypotheses and theories that made medicine an esoteric topic. And the demystifying of medicine could only be to the advantage of the masses, who were excluded from participating in their own healing because the physicians bombarded them with "technical terms, utterly unintelligible" to plain men and women.[16]

In seeking a "primitive" physic, Wesley sought a return to a "traditional" method of medical practice. He believed that early medicine, like early religion, had been "chiefly traditional," handed over from generation to generation and altered through experience and experiment. The demise of that tradition had begun when the learned started setting experience aside and building medical knowledge upon hypotheses and theories. The theories had led to the disregard of simple cures, substituting for them an abundance of "compound medicines" that often contained dangerous chemicals.[17]

Wesley's argument for simplicity had three practical consequences. He eliminated such "herculean" medicines as opium, steel, bark (which contained the chemical components of quinine), and most preparations made from quicksilver. In their place he substituted such simple prescriptions as fresh air, fresh water, small beer, honey, and herbs, along with a few "foreign medicines." He eliminated expensive medicines, thereby making cures available to the poor. And he altered medicine's preoccupation with illness by shifting its attention to health. Wesley urged careful attention to diet and exercise, rest and equanimity, temperance and cleanliness.[18]

In the meantime, people were sick. Wesley prescribed the best simple medication he knew. To a modern reader, his solutions provide delightful—and comical—entertainment. For fevers, he recommended tartar salt or sulphur spirits or cold baths. He urged persons suffering from St. Anthony's fire, a fever with painful swelling and blisters, to drink tar-water or sea-water or a "decoction of elder leaves, for a sweat." For "an easy and safe vomit," he recommended warm water flavored with artichoke leaves or radish seed. For baldness, the solution was daily applications of onions

and honey. Simple lunacy could be cured, he thought, by herbs or electricity. A raging madness, though, might require one to sit under a waterfall
or eat only apples for a month.[19]

The prescriptions, one must remember, came from standard books of
medical advice. Physicians and apothecaries made the same kinds of suggestions. They recommended pills made from dried and powdered toads,
ointments made from frog sperm, and decoctions from sheep's milk. Sir
Robert Boyle of the Royal Society provided Wesley with the suggestion
that the powder of mushroom puff-balls would stop bleeding and that the
yeast of beer would remove corns. Wesley's book was distinctive only in its
hesitation to recommend extreme solutions like bleeding or purges.[20]

His chief principle of good health, however, Wesley derived from the
story of the Fall in the book of Genesis. "In the sweat of thy face shalt thou
eat bread," God said, "till thou return to the ground." Because Wesley
considered God to be merciful, he could not consider the passage simply as
punitive, and its restorative intent he found in the reference to sweat. Both
Scripture and experience therefore taught him that "the power of exercise
both to preserve and restore health, is greater than will be conceived." And
Wesley generalized the admonition to exercise into a broader principle of
human health that he called "regimen."[21]

Regimen meant physical exercise. Wesley constantly returned to the
theme; he recommended at least two hours of walking or horseback riding
every day. He advised friends who were ill to take ample exercise in the
fresh air. And he attempted to explain the benefits of exercise so that the
grounds of his admonitions would be obvious to all. The body, he thought,
consisted of earth, air, fire, and water. To maintain the supply of water
and fire, the lungs had continually to take in air, which contained also par-
ticles of fire. The virtue of exercise was that it quickened the motion of the
lungs and enabled them to collect from the air a due amount of the fire,
which then radiated through the nerves. When the lungs diffused the fire
throughout the body, it became lively and vigorous; when the lungs failed
to accomplish their work ("which without exercise it cannot be"), the body
grew faint and languid.[22]

Regimen entailed more, though, than merely exercise. It meant the disciplining of physical life through careful attention to such matters as
cleanliness, diet, and sleep. Wesley thought that excessive sleep damaged
both body and mind. No man in good health, he said, should require more
than six or seven hours of sleep in twenty-four; no healthy woman should
require more than seven or eight. (Wesley believed that women were physically weaker.) Such moderation in sleeping habits Wesley found "prefer-

able to any medicine which I have known, both for preventing and removing nervous disorders."[23]

He thought that intemperance in food and drink slowly destroyed the body. Wesley's mother had insisted that her children eat sparingly, and when Wesley was a student at Oxford he found her intuitive wisdom confirmed by the studies of George Cheyne. Thereafter he tried to maintain a moderate diet. He avoided highly seasoned foods. He drank water and milk and limited amounts of wine and ale, and he abstained from all distilled liquors. He also abstained for years from tea, after he found at Oxford that it seemed to produce a mild paralytic disorder in his hand. For a while he drank weak tea, but eventually he left if off altogether for twelve years, resuming the use of it only when a physician whom he trusted recommended that he do so.[24]

Cleanliness promoted health, according to Wesley. He popularized among his Methodists the slogan "cleanliness is next to godliness," and he argued that the absence of hygiene was among the chief causes of disease. In eighteenth-century England, bathing was infrequent, and even the aristocrats who journeyed to Bath sought perfumes mainly to disguise the strong odor of their bodies and wore wigs partly to cover hair unwashed for months. In such a setting, Wesley seemed odd in recommending frequent cold baths, urging householders not to place their dung hills under their windows, telling Methodists to rid themselves of lice and bury their excrement, and advising them to avoid snuff and tobacco. But such safeguards were merely expressions of regimen.[25]

By no means, then, did Wesley believe that "all disease was due to demonism." He did think that all disease resulted ultimately from a primeval fall, but he believed that it resulted penultimately from unhealthy habits, hurtful chemicals, filthy environments, disproportionate emotions, and hereditary weakness. One of Wesley's few disagreements with William Cadogan's dissertation on gout was the physician's inattention to heredity. Cadogan emphasized intemperance; Wesley observed that he was temperate and nevertheless had suffered from gout; he believed that the reason lay in the fact that his mother had died from gout and his father had frequently been ill with it. Most diseases, and most cures, were, he thought, natural rather than supernatural.[26]

Wesley did hold that some diseases were of demonic origin and some cures were miraculous. Miraculous cures were works of omnipotence "wrought by the supernatural power of God." They were events "beyond the ordinary course of nature." Wesley admitted that "we do not know the precise bounds between nature and miracle." But he thought that miracles occurred, and that we could recognize them. And he believed in miracles of healing. Three doctors once told him that "there was but one method of cure" for an ailment from which he happened to be suffering. He demurred: "Perhaps but one natural one; but I think God has more than one method of healing either the soul or the body."[27]

Wesley once heard a doctor attribute a woman's fits to the malady that formerly had been called possession by a witch. He returned to his journal and angrily recorded the incident: "And why should they not call it so now. Because the infidels have hooted witchcraft out of the world, and the complaisant Christians, in large numbers, have joined with them in the cry." To Wesley it seemed that belief in witchcraft and the demonic had been presupposed throughout the New Testament. To abandon that belief, he feared, was to abandon the Bible.[28]

In Wesley's world angels and demons regularly made the passage from the supernatural world to the natural one. He always considered it possible that an episode of illness might be the work of satanic powers. "I can easily conceive, Satan will so disguise his part therein, that we cannot precisely determine, which part of the disorder is natural, and which preternatural." But Wesley tried to make that determination on more than one occasion. Once in 1764 he found a woman in a fit but judged it "plainly natural." Believing it to be epilepsy, he recommended electrical therapy. But on another occasion he ran across two women in distress, judged their malady to be demonic, and prayed for their delivery. He thought his prayer answered, but his Protestant critics accused him of "Romish exorcism." Yet in Wesley's world of thought and belief, devils could cause disease and angels could remove it, and something like exorcism seemed eminently plausible.[29]

Wesley would not have admitted to being an exorcist, and he also would never have referred to himself, in that setting, as a healer. He believed that certain persons might well be granted the extraordinary gifts of the Spirit, which included the gift of healing. But the healing was a gift from God, not an accomplishment of the healer. In explaining once how he had been healed of a painful sickness, Wesley emphasized that he had not expected the cure and did not look for such cures, because he believed that God did not intervene in accord with "the will" of men and women. Wesley expelled from the Methodist societies one George Bell who claimed the ability to cure with spittle and biblical formulas.[30]

But Wesley prayed for good health, both for himself and for others, and he believed that his prayers frequently were answered. Just as there had been healing miracles in the early church, so there were healing miracles, he thought, in the eighteenth century. He thought that prayer was especially necessary in cases of demonic possession. He once visited a young woman who first had suffered from depression and then had fallen into "utter distraction." He quickly decided that the physicians could not heal her, for the source of the disorder was supernatural: "This kind goeth not out but by prayer and fasting." When physicians could offer no rational account or effective remedy, Wesley was inclined to suspect evil spirits.[31]

Yet Wesley also prayed for healing when the source of the malady appeared to be strictly natural or organic. He believed in the possibility of supernatural cures, and he sought them. He prayed for a distracted woman and reported that she found instant relief; she was "restored to a sound mind." He prayed for a woman in bodily pain; she arose without pain the following day. He prayed while his brother suffered from pleurisy, and his brother was cured while Wesley was at prayer. He prayed for relief from his own acute pain; the pain disappeared. Wesley had no doubt that the recovery was a gift from a merciful God.[32]

He had no difficulty, therefore, accepting reports of other similar miraculous cures. One of his preachers prayed for a woman with a breast disease and reported that she had been cured. Wesley examined the case, and concluded that he was right: "1. She was ill. 2. She is well. 3. She became so in a moment. Which of these can with modesty be denied." He normally tried to account for seemingly miraculous healings by examining first the possible natural causes. But Wesley had little skepticism about reports of supernatural healing. And it is true that he once prayed for his horse when it was lame, with the result, he said, that the lameness immediately disappeared, and he and the horse continued on their journey.[33]

He also thought that piety itself was healing. The "love of God" was the sovereign remedy of all miseries, because it gave the mind serenity and tranquility. Piety could not preclude the possibility of sickness; Wesley thought that even the perfect Christian would have to bear the infirmities of the body. But the calm joy of faith nurtured the body, and the distress of emotional grief harmed it.[34] He did not assume, however, that the health which flowed from piety and the healing that came as a response to prayer were the same. He never tried to explain the healing efficacy of prayer by referring to its psychological benefits or by claiming that it conferred a healthy equanimity. Prayer for Wesley was a petition to God. And it was God, not prayer, he thought, who healed.[35]

Wesley therefore held in balance two perspectives on health and healing, one natural and one preternatural. In his mind the two never conflicted with each other, and he felt an intense curiosity about both of them. He never imagined that the balance could be lost or that the tension between the two visions could disrupt his Methodist movement. But by the mid-nineteenth century, the issue of health and healing became a point of severe contention within the Methodist churches.

## TRADITION: SPIRITUAL HEALING

During his lifetime, Wesley publicized the theme of spiritual healing by including in his *Arminian Magazine* assorted narratives of extraordinary cures. He turned even to the seventeenth century for examples of healings that occurred in response to prayer and faith.[36] After his death in 1791, class leaders continued to pray for the sick, and Methodists continued to hope for supernatural cures. But the interest in spiritual healing receded for a time.

Within four decades of Wesley's death, however, some of his successors were insisting that Methodism should promote spiritual healing. The insistence reflected in part a new effort to interpret the spiritual pilgrimage that Wesley had defined as typical of the Christian life—the movement from prevenient grace to entire sanctification. At the heart of the Methodist holiness crusade was the conviction that Wesley (and the Bible) expected the Christian to receive a distinctive gift of holiness as the result of a specifiable, supernatural work of grace subsequent to rebirth. The advocates of holiness spoke not of a gradual perfecting that lured the Christian into the future but of a "second blessing" that conferred the status of Christian perfection. By accenting the suddenness of the experience, they minimized Wesley's emphasis on a gradual process of growth, which had provided the doctrinal setting for his own understanding of Christian perfection.

The holiness movement within Methodism was one expression of a broader interest in the doctrine of sanctification in America and England. Among Methodists it emerged in the late 1830s, when Sarah Lankford and Phoebe Palmer of New York City organized a weekly prayer session which became widely known as the Tuesday Meeting. The movement soon had its own influential journal, *The Guide to Holiness*, and by the 1840s began to attract support within the denomination for its insistence on the necessity of a crisis experience and a public testimony about it.

During the 1850s the proponents of a specifiable "second blessing" of entire holiness spoke increasingly of an activity of the Holy Spirit which endued the faithful Christian with power. In 1856 the Irish Methodist William Arthur published *The Tongue of Fire*, a popular book which intensified expectations about the work of the Spirit, both in America and in the British Isles. When Phoebe Palmer toured Britain during the 1860s, she reported dramatic outbreaks of revivalist fervor, which she and other Methodist revivalists began to interpret as the return of the spiritual power of the first Pentecost, a time when "many wonders and signs were done through the apostles" (Acts 2:1–47).

Wesleyans therefore were leaders in organizing in America during the 1860s National Camp Meetings to promote holiness as well as a National Association for the Promotion of Holiness. The holiness camp meetings engendered an ecstatic revivalist piety, a heightened sense of expectancy about the supernatural activity of the Spirit, and a growing interest in the "extraordinary" gifts of the Spirit, which included the gift of healing. When the president of the Association, the Methodist John Inskip, reported in 1871 that he had received divine healing for ailments that had resulted from sunstroke, the "healing question" began to be troubling.[37]

Methodists in England and America debated the question of healing in 1872, when the British physicist John Tyndall endorsed a Prayer Test to verify, or expose, assertions about spiritual healing. Tyndall suggested that a single hospital ward be designated as a laboratory of divine healing in which objective observers could judge whether prayer had any significant influence on the recovery of the sick. The response from British Methodists was mixed. Some thought that the project would constitute a presumptuous testing of God; some thought it unwarrantable interference with destiny; others favored it.

In America the reaction was similar. A prayer of that kind, wrote one Methodist, would be "mere magical incantation." No prayer uttered with "one eye faintly resting on the hospital, the other intently scanning the medical world" could properly be considered Christian prayer, in any case. But other American Methodists thought it an exciting proposal. The conflicting reactions revealed the potential disagreements within the tradition.[38]

Affirmations of spiritual healing had long elicited considerable credence and interest in America. The African slaves, acting in accord with traditional conceptions of healing by diviners and conjurers, had constituted a large subculture in which nonphysical means of healing were widely practiced. Confidence in divine healing extended also to white churches. As early as 1846, one Ethan O. Allen had persuaded reluctant Methodist class leaders to pray that he might be healed of consumption, and his prompt recovery encouraged him to launch a career as an itinerant faith healer; a number of Methodists found his message appealing, even when his *Faith Healing* (1881) carried the Wesleyan doctrine of perfection to its physical extreme by arguing that purification from sin would eliminate illness.[39]

In the nascent healing movement, Allen was a minor figure compared to Charles Cullis, an Episcopalian physician from Boston who became swept up in the piety of the holiness crusade after attending one of Phoebe Palmer's Tuesday Meetings. Upon reading the biography of a Swiss healer named Dorothea Trudel, Cullis began in 1870 to practice spiritual healing, and it was he who convinced a few prominent Methodists, including Inskip and Daniel Steele, a professor at Boston University, that full salvation included not only the healing of the spirit but also the healing of the body.[40] Cullis was popular among holiness Methodists, and he conducted at Methodist campgrounds in New England a number of gatherings for healing services. He also found Methodist allies who defended his views in the denomination's churches and conventions. One contributor to the influential *Christian Advocate* in New York used Cullis's movement as the occasion to boast that "believing prayer is as efficacious in America as in England."[41]

But the proponents of healing also aroused resistance. The leader of the resistance was a New York minister named James M. Buckley, editor of the *Advocate*. As early as 1875, Buckley addressed the Methodist preachers of New York and told them that faith healing was "a kind of quackery of faith." In his *Address on Supposed Miracles* (1875), he insisted that the pretense of spiritual healing degraded faith to the level of superstition, and in the three decades between 1880 and 1912, he conducted a relentless campaign against the "absurdity" of faith healing, which he thought to be an irrational and magical attempt to control God. Buckley acknowledged that nonmedical healings might occur, but he insisted that they simply exhibited the psychological efficacy of confident belief, that they occurred in other religions and in secular settings, and that they had nothing to do with true Christian trust. The New Testament, he said, "teaches that the highest good is the knowledge and love of God, and that the Spirit of God has constant access to the minds of men, and sets forth an all-inclusive doctrine of Providence without whom not even a sparrow falls. It does not say that prayer will always secure the recovery of the sick."[42]

Other writers in the *Christian Advocate* claimed that the mission of Christianity was to the soul, not to the body, and they urged the ministers of the denomination not to turn Christian faith into a substitute for patent medicines. They attributed spiritual healing to the "effects of imagination and excitement" and suggested that the era of healing miracles had ended with the advance of education and science.[43]

The advocates of healing replied that no belief was "rising more swiftly before the churches everywhere than that of Divine Healing." They attributed opposition to a naturalistic bias against the miraculous; they insisted that the ministry of Jesus had included the healing of the body; they argued that the doctrine of creation affirmed the goodness of the body; and they argued that entire sanctification had to encompass our whole life as embodied creatures. They also quoted at length from John Wesley's journals. And, being Methodists, they sang their faith: "Standing on the promises of Christ my King, / Through eternal ages let his praises ring; / Standing on the promises of God."[44]

Increasingly, though, the proponents both of the "second blessing" and of healing began to leave the Methodist church and join smaller groups, some of them Wesleyan in origin, in which divine healing attracted more intense support. In the Pilgrim Holiness and Wesleyan Methodist and Free Methodist churches, the advocates of healing felt more at home. A number of other Wesleyans became caught up in the Pentecostal fervor that erupted after 1901 when Charles Parham, a one-time Methodist evangelist, helped convince the students of Bethel Bible College in Kansas that the primary sign of the indwelling of the Spirit was the ability to speak in tongues. Parham had been attracted to the healing crusade of Alexander Dowie in Zion City, Illinois, and he helped to ensure that a preoccupation with faith healing would be a central feature of the Penecostal churches that began to form after 1906. After William J. Seymour's tumultuous revival at the Azusa Street Church in Los Angeles in 1906, both Pentecostal fervor and a devout trust in spiritual healing began to permeate a segment of Wesleyan churches, black and white, especially those within lower-scale economic groups.[45]

The interest in spiritual healing did not disappear in the larger middle-class Methodist denominations. In England, especially, the resurgence of interest in psychology after the First World War led a significant body of English Methodists to explore the possibilities once again. But the attention to healing among the twentieth-century English Methodists did not assume belief in a supernatural "second blessing" of entire holiness. Their exploration of spiritual healing represented an effort to disengage the notion of nonphysical healing from the vision of the Christian journey that had been popular among holiness Wesleyans in nineteenth-century America. The proponents of healing in England understood the journey as a gradual development toward higher levels of Christian insight and maturity. But they believed that their vision of the journey, informed now by depth psychology and psychosomatic medicine, also required that they attend to the ministry of healing.

As a chaplain in the war, the English Methodist Leslie Weatherhead decided that "to relegate all healing to the medical methods of the doctors, splendid though that work is, did not really answer the challenges of our Lord's words." Determined to learn all he could about nonphysical means of cure, he joined a study group of doctors and ministers who took turns each week introducing and discussing a new book on health and healing. Weatherhead concluded that the Christian Church had lost its secret of spiritual healing and that the new psychology offered a way to regain it.[46]

Through regular articles on psychology in the *Methodist Recorder*, Weatherhead drew attention to his use of psychotherapeutic methods in his own parish. In 1936 he took those methods to City Temple in London, where he established close working relationships with physicians by establishing a psychological clinic in the church. In the same year he presented to the Methodist Conference the report of a Committee on Spiritual Healing that he had chaired. He prefaced his report by saying that the first task of the Church was to bring people into a vital relationship with God and that the question of health must remain always subordinate to that aim. But he proposed that Methodist theological students be introduced to clinical psychology, that churches set up experimental clinics in which doctors and ministers might cooperate, and that intercessory prayer for the sick be encouraged throughout the Methodist church. The proposal did not meet with universal approval, but Weatherhead hoped to avoid the divisiveness that had troubled American Methodists. He would seek to restore Wesley's sense of the harmony between therapeutic medicine and spiritual healing.[47]

Alongside his counseling and his work with the doctors at the City Temple Clinic, therefore, he continued a practice that he had begun at his parish in Leeds: weekly periods of directed intercessory prayer in the congregation. "Don't think that you are trying to persuade a reluctant God to heal the sufferer," he would tell his praying congregation. "And don't pray that he may become better, for that is to put his cure in the future. But imagine you are bringing him into the presence of Christ and that Christ is laying his hands on him. Believe that at this moment the healing power is working."[48]

He thought that some miraculous healings had resulted from the services, but he was modest in his claims. In fewer than 5 percent of the cases could he be confident that the prayers had been followed by discernible improvement. He acknowledged that even in those instances the evidence would not have convinced a skeptical critic. Weatherhead himself remained skeptical about most claims of spiritual healing. In his *Psychology, Religion and Healing* (1951), he concluded that pitifully few healings occurred at Lourdes, that the healings claimed by Christian Scientists were largely accidental, and that dramatic healing missions in large assemblies were manipulative and misleading. But he did believe that the prayers of faithful Christians could constitute a ministry of "spiritual healing" because Christ had possessed a supernatural gift of healing, and because the Church, as the extension of Christ's incarnation, could in its corporate life appropriate that spiritual power.[49]

Weatherhead won considerable support from English Methodists. "Prayer, with intent to cure physical ailment, is, to say the least of it, not presumptuous," wrote one of his supporters. Through the Methodist Committee on Healing which he helped to form, the denomination in England launched a study of healing and health in the New Testament, the early church, and modern England. One result of the study was the formation in 1946 of the Methodist Society for Medical and Pastoral Practice, an organization to promote closer alliances between ministers and doctors and also to explore the possibilities of spiritual healing. The society affirmed that "health of body, mind and spirit is the will of God, and that illness of any kind belongs to the kingdom of evil, and should be attacked." It denied that suffering could be considered a "condition of saintliness."[50]

The secretary of the society, John Crowlesmith, believed that the eighteenth-century Methodist revival had properly been occupied with matters "deeper and more important" than religious healing, but he also thought that the Church's practice of spiritual healing had preserved Jesus' conception of God as the compassionate One who sought the good of men and women, not their suffering or misfortune. The position of the society was one of unreserved support for medical science. But the members were also convinced that "the art of healing does not lie only within the province of orthodox medicine."[51]

The English Methodists in the Society for Medical and Pastoral Practice felt suspicious of the claims that some nineteenth-century Americans had seemed to make on behalf of faith healing. In 1962 the society published some of the conclusions that its members had reached after sixteen years of study, conferences, and discussion. Their publication, *Religion and Medicine*, reflected no consensus. It did reflect a wariness about faith healers. One New Testament scholar warned that the Bible did not "provide us with a technique of healing which will be valid for all time" and suggested that modern faith healers might be attempting an unintelligent imitation of the New Testament grounded in a superficial interpretation of Christianity. "Faith," he said, "must be rescued from the faith-healers." The word of faith in the New Testament proclaimed that "God was in the situation, however incurable the disease seemed to be, or however the demoniac raved."[52]

Similar warnings appeared throughout the volume. The theologian William Strawson observed that the mention of spiritual healing commonly elicited images of eccentric cranks who failed to accept the discipline of a scientific method and who made unjustifiable claims. The biblical scholar Ronald Spivey insisted that in the Christian understanding all healing came from God, and he argued that the faith healers went astray at two junctures. First, their rhetoric about faith healing implied that the cure was a result of the faith, whereas Christians understood all healing as a gift of grace, not an accomplishment of faith. Second, their sharp separation between the natural and the supernatural reflected a faulty doctrine of God. "Everything that happens," he said, "happens naturally if God is the Creator and Ruler of nature." Even Weatherhead, who continued to hold intercessory services for the sick, acknowledged that if the value of intercessory prayer were to be judged "by its success as a means of making sick people well, we should be obliged to discontinue it," for "usually it makes no appreciable difference in the physical condition of the patient."[53]

Weatherhead continued to believe, however, that in some instances prayer for recovery seemed effective, and he hoped that "the rare occasions when healing follows and seems to be due to prayer should be relentlessly examined." Strawson also thought that prayer might be a means of drawing on divine resources of healing: "When he prays, the Christian is not expecting God to alter His plans for the future; he is bringing to God the factor of his interest and obedience, in the conviction that these will contribute to the way events will develop in the future." The emerging consensus was that healing might well follow prayer, but that the matter lay beyond proof and calculation. Increasingly, moreover, the Methodist pastors in the Society for Medical and Pastoral Practice found it awkward to interpret spiritual healing as an appeal to a supernatural realm that stood in contrast to the realm of natural experience. Their tendency was rather to expand the meaning of the natural so as to recognize the extent to which it allowed for unexpected possibilities. They believed that all healing came from God, but they tended to view natural events not in contrast to divine acts but in the context of the divine reality, so that if "through spiritual means a cure is effected, this is only a farther instance of the same healing power which might have been used through medicine if only the right method had been known."[54]

In popular English Methodism, an interest in spiritual healing has remained an undercurrent of piety. Such exponents of healing as Elsie Salmon have periodically conducted quiet healing services in Methodist churches whose members believed that prayers for the healing of the body reflected a Christian commitment to the wholeness of the person.[55]

In America, as well, a few Methodist congregations have sponsored services of healing, and a few ministers have remained committed to the possibility. Despite the earlier tensions in American Methodism, a survey of American Methodist ministers in 1954 revealed that 29 percent had "attempted to perform a spiritual healing." By 1965 at least twenty Methodist churches in the United States—out of about forty thousand local congregations—were holding regular healing services. An example was the First United Methodist Church of Collingswood, New Jersey, whose minister, Frank Stanger (by 1960 the president of Asbury Theological Seminary), explained his interest in a ministry of healing as a renewed quest for "total ministry" to the "whole person." Accepting Leslie Weatherhead's definition of healing as "the process of restoring the broken harmony which prevents personality, at any point of body, mind, or spirit, from its perfect functioning," Stanger insisted that Jesus' commission to his disciples made a healing ministry mandatory for the Church. It fulfilled that mandate by inspiring healthy living, creating healthy attitudes, cooperating with physicians and surgeons, understanding psychosomatic illness, and praying for God's intervention. And it could do so because the creative God willed wholeness, not suffering, for the created order. Stanger therefore arranged services consisting of testimonies, prayers of healing, and intercessions.[56]

Another well-known example was the New Life Clinic conducted by Albert E. Day in a Methodist congregation in Baltimore. Day made no claim to be a healer. "It is God who heals," he said. He acknowledged that his efforts often failed: "We do not attempt to conceal or explain away any failures." He was careful to insist that his healing ministry sought God as an end, not as a means to a lesser end. But by silent prayer and laying on of hands, in the midst of a congregation silently at prayer, Day conducted a "ministry of silence" that sought health and healing for the sick.[57]

Day did not describe himself as a healer, but some of his allies seemed less circumspect. Olga and Ambrose Worrall, who began their lay ministry of spiritual healing under Day's direction, felt free to define the spiritual qualities required in the "healer," as well as the spiritual capacities required of the "patient." Their emphasis fell on the intensity of the patient's "belief." The implication was that healing could occur through the accomplishments of gifted healers and faithful patients who lived and believed in accord with "natural laws" of health.[58]

Like many other healers, the Worralls reflected the influence of a tradition outside historic Methodism: New Thought. In the New Thought traditions, which had their American origins in the healing methods of Phineas Quimby in the 1840s, healing issued from the mind's capacity to entertain ideas and attitudes that enabled it to tap resources of power immanent within the self and the world. New Thought and Wesleyanism represented two distinctive visions of God and the self.

In the Wesleyan tradition, healing was an undeserved gift; in the New Thought tradition, healing was an accomplishment achieved through careful mastery of one's own mind and disposition. In the Wesleyan tradition, spiritual healing was a mystery, utterly beyond calculation; in the New Thought tradition, the conditions requisite for successful healing could be stipulated. In the early Wesleyan tradition, healing was incidental to wider aims; in New Thought, other aims were incidental to the end of healing.

Some of the interest in spiritual healing within modern Methodism, in short, represents a blending of two incompatible traditions. When one insists that "practically all the diseases and infirmities that science has not conquered are emotionally induced" and employs that highly doubtful assumption as an explanation for miracles of healing, one has combined scientific error and religious shallowness. The truth is that we have precious little reliable insight into the emotional component of serious illness, and that we can hardly justify the concept of the miraculous by reducing it to the status of a category in psychosomatic medicine. When one insists that "healing will follow" if the conditions of obedience to the "law of spiritual health" are met, one loses sight of Wesley's intense struggle with the dialectic of law and gospel. Interpretations of that sort reflect an appropriation of New Thought categories within the Methodist tradition.[59]

In the United States, of course, the public often associates faith healing primarily with celebrated faith healers, and for one brief period none was more widely celebrated than Oral Roberts, who began his career as a minister of the Pentecostal Holiness Church, a denomination with Wesleyan roots. Claiming that he himself had been healed of stuttering and tuberculosis by a revivalist healer, Roberts insisted that God had endowed his right hand with the "healing virtue of the Son of God." He eventually established a vast organization called Healing Waters and during the 1950s extended his appeal through vivid televised healing services. The enterprise grew through the sale and distribution of magazines, tracts, books, prayer cloths, and holy oil. Thousands stood in prayer lines in Roberts's tent, awaiting his prayer and the "point of contact" with his right hand.[60]

In 1968 Roberts joined the United Methodist Church and soon ended his healing crusades, devoting most of his time to a university he had founded in Tulsa, Oklahoma. He resumed his earlier preoccupation with healing when in 1978 he opened a medical school at the university and broke ground for a hospital complex which he called a City of Faith. In his hospitals he hoped to combine the benefits of scientific medicine and spiritual healing.[61]

Prayer for healing is clearly compatible with the Methodist tradition. It could hardly be otherwise, for Wesley recognized that prayer was no mere verbal formulation. Prayer, for Wesley, referred to the deepest disposition of the self toward God. For that reason, he could instruct his Methodists repeatedly to "pray without ceasing." And as the reflection of the self's depths, prayer must inevitably bear within it a plea for the good of the beloved.

Yet Wesley never designated himself as a special agent of healing, never made healing central to his revival, never conducted healing services, and never found in the biblical stories specifiable rules for healing. He believed in the possibility of healing as a response to prayer, but he wrote little about it and preached about it hardly at all. Wesley's vision had a different center; spiritual healing lay at the periphery.

Spiritual healing has never been a central theme for the Methodist movement. Recognizing that their confidence in a merciful and mysterious God always permitted trust in a possibility beyond our limited possibilities, the Methodist churches have nevertheless shown little interest in a piety which moves that trust in divine healing to the forefront of the religious life. Such a piety has remained on the periphery of the tradition, just as it remained peripheral to Wesley's revival in eighteenth-century England.

## TRADITION: HEALTH

Most Methodists have found other ways to reflect on health and healing, ways more in keeping with a vision of the Christian journey as a gradual development from sinfulness to holiness, from fragmentation to wholeness. They have valued the Wesley who cured the physical body because he recognized its unity with the soul, who urged regimen and discipline of the recalcitrant flesh, or who recognized that stomach pain could result from grief as well as from ulcers. They have found those visions of health and healing to be congruent with a broader vision of Christian life as a gradual and grace-filled passage through an uncharted future.

The images of health have changed through the years. Wesley thought of health as one dimension of human wholeness. Throughout the century after Wesley's death in 1791, Methodists who attended to matters of health and healing viewed health mainly as the absence of impairment. By 1891, however, they viewed it from a different, more optimistic, more ebullient perspective. They saw it not simply as the absence of impairment but as the positive capacity to maintain and enhance physical function. And by the time another fifty years had passed, they were thinking in yet more expansive terms, defining—or presupposing a vision of—health as the harmonious functioning of a unified person within a community of other persons.

The early Methodists, despite their deep sense of corporate piety, normally spoke of health and healing with a highly individualistic vocabulary. They viewed illness as the impairment of specific functions, and the Wesley whom they found most useful as a guide in matters of illness and health was the Wesley who wrote the *Primitive Physick*.

Physical health was not for them, however, a goal or criterion of religious faith. Richard Watson, the great English systematician of early Wesleyan doctrine, expressed a typical early Methodist attitude when he wrote in his *Theological Institutes* (1823) that "it is more our duty to obey God than to take care of our health and life." His sentiment suggested no disdain for good health. A physically fragile man who suffered from chronic illness and pain almost all his adult life, Watson could exhort his daughter to "walk much in the garden" for the sake of her health. But health was for him less important than piety. To be ill was to suffer for a time; to be impious was to suffer for eternity.[62]

Like Watson, other early Methodists subordinated physical health to spiritual wholeness, but the movement did not neglect the body. In the waning years of the eighteenth century and the early years of the nineteenth, Wesleyan preachers still dispensed medical prescriptions. On the American frontier, where Methodism became one of the largest of the Protestant churches in the United States, the circuit riders—preachers who rode horseback to visit the Methodist societies in their region—were often the closest approximation to a physician that anyone could find. Some Methodist preachers took that fact seriously. James Gilruth, a traveling preacher in the Ohio Conference in 1831, for example, was doing nothing unusual when he "visited Br. Wm. Brown, a local [Preacher] now living in this Neighborhood . . . and spent a couple of hours quite agreeably conversing principly on the study of Medicine in which he is now engaged having furnished himself with a pretty good Medical Library." Circuit riders brought not only the gospel but also medicines and suggestions for home remedies.[63]

Wesley's *Primitive Physick* continued to find a wide audience. Between 1791 and 1881, the book went through more than forty-five editions. In America it was published under the auspices of the new Methodist Episcopal Church. But Methodists in England were, if anything, more enthusiastic than their American counterparts. By the end of the nineteenth century one could count at least thirty-eight English editions of the book, as compared to twenty-four editions in America.[64]

The publication of the book proceeded despite a growing accommodation between preachers and physicians. Doctors had been critical of Wesley's prescriptions, and he had been critical of theirs. But it was of symbolic importance that a physician preached Wesley's funeral sermon, for as Methodism began to expand into the middle classes of England and America, doctors began to feel at home in the movement. By the early nineteenth century, some of Wesley's harsher criticisms of doctors and drugs seemed to some Methodists to have been insufficiently thoughtful.[65]

When the leaders of American Methodism, Thomas Coke and Francis Asbury, decided in the 1790s that it would be useful to reprint the *Primitive Physick* for Americans, they turned for help to physicians. Because food and climate were different in America, they thought that Wesley's book should be "revised by physicians practicing in this country." They requested that the doctors add "cautionary notes when they are necessary," as well as provide "additional receipts suitable to the climate." The doctors proved more than willing to append their revisions.[66] The preachers asked Dr. Henry Wilkins, a graduate of the Medical College of the University of Pennsylvania, to assume primary responsibility for the revision, and he promptly turned to other standard medical works for additional insight. By the time his work was completed, Wilkins had compiled his own vast collection of medical remedies. Rather than radically alter Wesley's list, he chose to publish the two sets of recommendations under one title, *The Family Advisor* (1793), with his own medical suggestions prominently located at the front of the volume.

As an admirer of the American physician Benjamin Rush, whose work at the University of Pennsylvania suggested that all disease resulted from excessive or convulsive actions of the arteries, Wilkins had a special fondness for the remedy of which Wesley had been most suspicious: bleeding. Coke and Asbury still believed that "simple remedies are, in general, the most safe for simple disorders." But Wilkins attended to a host of unsafe disorders, as well, and he recommended Rush's "heroic" measures. Inflammation of the brain, for example, required bleeding, more bleeding, and then more bleeding. A careful reader could easily have wondered whether Wilkins and Wesley belonged under the same cover.[67]

In one respect, Wesley and Wilkins proceeded in the same manner. They listed isolated ailments, one by one, and suggested specific remedies for each. Wesley had believed that the individual ailments resulted from a disruption of the whole person, and he had remained sensitive to the interrelatedness of the soul and the body. But when Methodists republished the *Primitive Physick*, they had no way of setting its isolated recommendations within Wesley's broader theological understanding of bodies and souls. The result was that the book encouraged a negative conception of health as the simple absence of impairment, and it conceived of impairment as the malfunctioning of specific organs and systems of the body. Wesley had been deeply aware of the possible connections between, say, pain in the stomach and grief in the heart, but he had not expounded that awareness in the *Primitive Physick*. The continued publication of the book, torn from its larger theological context, entailed, therefore, a diminution of Wesley's insight.

The Methodist classes, however, did maintain something of Wesley's stress on the importance of systematically visiting the sick. The guides for class leaders still recommended both visits and prayers. One hardly knows how avidly the middle-class Methodists of Victorian England and Jacksonian America pursued their rounds among the sick, but the duty of caring for them remained a part of the Wesleyan tradition.

On more than one occasion, an instance of caring has become part of the self-understanding of one or another Methodist group. The African Methodist Episcopal Church, a black denomination which began in protest against white discrimination in the eighteenth century, retains as part of its heritage a dramatic account of visits to the sick and dying during the epidemic of yellow fever in Philadelphia in 1793. Richard Allen, founder of the church and also its first bishop, included in the record of his "life experience and gospel labors" a narrative of the epidemic and of his ministry within it. Because white physicians believed blacks to be immune to the infection, they requested their help in caring for the dying and burying the dead. Allen knew that a positive reply brought a risk, but he and his friends decided, after prayer, that it was their "duty to do all the good we could to our suffering fellow mortals."[68]

Allen spent days removing the dead, procuring nurses, and offering medical services. At the request of Benjamin Rush, he administered medicine and bled the seriously ill. "We were willing to imitate the doctor's benevolence, who, sick or well, kept his house open day and night, to give what assistance he could in this time of trouble." He wrote his narrative account primarily to answer critics who charged that blacks had profited from the suffering; it revealed that he had not only healed the sick and cared for the dying but had also paid for their coffins with his own money. Thus a moment of medical care became a part of the African Methodist Episcopal tradition, and of the wider Methodist tradition as well.[69]

The early Methodists viewed health and piety as intertwined, with health always in the subordinate position. Whether they sought prescriptions in medical guidebooks or devoted themselves to visiting the sick, they acted within a setting of revivalist piety and evangelical fervor. Among the African slaves in the American South, illness provided an occasion for the joining of African tradition and evangelical piety. The slaves relied on traditional herbal medication and sought the aid of "conjure doctors" who healed with spells and charms, but they viewed such practices and practitioners through eyes that had been opened to the delights of ecstatic, revivalist Methodism. Among the middle-class Methodists of English and American cities, on the other hand, illness provided an occasion for the joining of Victorian moralism and evangelical piety. These Methodists assured each other that to seek health was to fulfill the duty of "physical culture," an ingredient in the broader spiritual disciplining of mature Christians.[70]

The temptation of Christians has always been to baptize cultural goods and then to claim them as the fruits of Christian piety. To nineteenth-century Methodists, such a temptation proved irresistible. Preoccupied with demonstrating the credibility of their faith, they soon found themselves arguing that medicine owed its successes to the Christian revelation. "A Christian civilization alone prizes human life," wrote a nineteenth-century Methodist journalist. "This also is the true basis of the healing art." Only the Christian faith could render the medical profession a necessity, for only "the spirit of Christ" could animate a constant care for "human life in all its stages, from conception to death." From the plausible premise that Christian faithfulness could issue in a benevolent care for physical well-being, Methodists sometimes proceeded to the doubtful—and self-serving—conclusion that the concern for physical well-being in Christian nations demonstrated the truth and superiority of the Christian faith.[71] Such arguments became especially popular in the late nineteenth century, when English Methodists became respectable and American Methodists became their nation's largest Protestant denomination.

By that time, Methodists had begun to expand not only their numbers but also their vision of health and medicine. Whereas their predecessors had viewed health as an absence of impairment, Methodists in the 1880s began to understand it as a positive capacity to maintain and enhance physical function. They gave increasing emphasis to images of muscular vitality and tonic self-mastery. Though retaining much of the older individualism, they became increasingly sensitive to the capacity of social institutions to advance or retard the physical well-being among larger groups of people. Though tending still to think of illness as the impairment of specific functions, they exhibited far greater interest in the environmental causes of illness and therefore in the interconnections of bodily functions. The Wesley whom they valued was the Wesley who had called for regimen as a solution to physical complaint and for service as an expression of spiritual growth.

The change reflected, in part, the economic transitions of the industrial revolution, which compelled the churches to recognize the power of social institutions. By the end of the nineteenth century, Methodists in England, America, and Europe had embarked on a course that would lead them to the forefront of the social gospel. The change also reflected Western culture's growing regard for physical and mental vitality. The late nineteenth century was an era in which popular philosophers talked about the power of the will and the strenuous mood, popularizers of Darwinian evolution talked about force and vitality within the cosmic process, popularizers of rugby and football advertised the moral value of sport, politicians boasted of imperial power and duty, and popularizers of piety began to preach about "muscular Christianity." Metaphors of power and service appeared across a broad spectrum of Christians in Europe and America, from holiness groups seeking power for service to social reformers seeking to serve the powerless.

Methodist rhetoric during the 1890s echoed that admiration for vitality. Methodists began to insist that because Christianity was "the religion of the body as well as of the soul," it should never be considered "a morbid and gloomy asceticism, [or] a namby-pamby sentimentality." "Its sainthood," wrote one bishop, "is not necessarily weak-chested and flabby-muscled." Its highest saints, even those who, like Paul the Apostle, seemed to suffer from physical infirmity, somehow possessed "a physical organization of extraordinary vigor and elasticity." Had Paul lived in our day, the bishop added, "he would have been no enemy to the gymnasium, or to the college boating club, or to any of the means of judicious physical culture with which the youth of this generation are favored."[72]

The rhetoric now seems quaint, but in the nineteenth century it seemed not only to represent a salutary protest against an earlier cult of sentimentality, which had viewed physical infirmity as a sign of piety, but also to suggest, in a popular phrase of the period, "new avenues of Christian service." All the talk about power and vitality found expression in a call for young Christians to throw themselves earnestly into the struggle against suffering, illness, poverty, and oppression. It was within such a setting of social responsibility that Methodists recovered the tradition of training deaconesses to serve both in hospitals and in the homes of the poor.[73]

In 1908 the Methodist Episcopal Church in the United States adopted a "Social Creed" that committed them to serve human need wherever it could be found. The social principles affirmed ideals of health: the regulation of working conditions, the provision of protection and recreation for children, and the safeguarding of workers from dangerous machinery, unsanitary working conditions, injuries, and occupational diseases. They insisted both on appropriate leisure and on the regulation of labor conditions for women. The Methodists called on Christians to recognize the golden rule and the mind of Christ "as the supreme law of society."[74]

In England the call for a social Christianity elicited a response especially from a talented Welshman named Hugh Price Hughes, whose sermons and editorial on "the Nonconformist Conscience" helped to turn English Methodists from political indifference and conservatism to active support for political reform and the Liberal Party. And the Methodist social gospel in England included a "gospel of health." To social liberals like Hughes it seemed certain that "when human society is reconstructed on a Christian basis, infant mortality and blighting disease will be mere memories of the buried past." The promise of the kingdom of God included a promise of bodily health, and it inspired a confidence that "disease is an avoidable and a removable evil." Hughes called on Methodists to "attack physical disease with all the resources of Christian civilization," especially by attending to its prevention through measures of public health. Hughes wanted to see parks in the cities, gymnasiums and free lunches in the schools, sanitary legislation in Parliament, pure water in the cities, and public-spirited honesty in the giant food markets.[75]

Enthusiasm for a social gospel undergirded the Methodist campaign to build hospitals as means of service, especially to the poor. Methodists had begun as early as 1787 to organize "Strangers' Friend Societies" to help "poor, sick, friendless strangers," and as early as 1790 an Association of Friends of the Sick Poor succeeded in building, in Waterford, Ireland, a fever hospital. But the movement lacked resources, so it was not until the late nineteenth century that Methodists began to invest heavily in the construction of hospitals.

In 1881, James Monroe Buckley, editor of the New York *Christian Advocate,* lamented that the Methodist Episcopal Church was "without a hospital [or] a dispensary." One of Buckley's parishioners had once died after an accident because no hospital was available, and the minister vowed from that moment to secure the erection of a Methodist hospital. When he became an editor, he sought to fulfill his vow. Having discovered that Saint Luke's Hospital in New York had cared for more than eight hundred Methodist patients, most of whom could not pay for the care, he determined that Methodists should at least be willing to reciprocate for such kindly deeds. He did not believe, he wrote in 1881, that the lack of Methodist hospitals resulted from any "unfriendly conviction." The problem was the "outcome of a preoccupation; but is it now time that somewhere we build a hospital?"[76]

When a wealthy New York layman, George I. Seney, read the editorial, he arranged a conversation with Buckley, who complained that Methodism seemed unconcerned about the suffering sick. Seney responded with a proposal: "I offer you sixteen eligible lots, valued at $40,000, as a site, and $100,000 in cash toward the erection of a Methodist Episcopal General Hospital, which shall be open to Jew and Gentile, Protestant and Catholic, heathen and infidel, on the same terms." He subsequently expanded his offer to include an entire city block and $200,000. The result of the conversation was the founding in 1881 of a denominational hospital in Brooklyn, New York, the first of an extended chain of Methodist hospitals throughout the world.[77]

The hospital in New York opened in 1887; the next year saw the opening of Wesley Hospital in Chicago. Within another two years, Methodists opened a hospital in Cincinnati; in 1892 they completed the Methodist hospitals in Philadelphia and Minneapolis. During the first half-century after the opening of their first institution, the Methodists built fifty-nine hospitals in the United States, and dozens in overseas missions.[78]

One can hardly explain the flurry of construction without recalling the rise of lay philanthropy among affluent Methodists in the mid-nineteenth century in America. Having once considered themselves as people of humble origins, they recognized after the Civil War that their membership now included a professional and commercial elite. When Bishop Matthew Simpson prepared in 1878 his *Cyclopaedia of Methodism*, he included 347 entries about influential laity, most of whom were listed because of their achievements in business and the professions. Those successful laypersons increasingly assumed positions of authority in the denomination; the church looked to them for both gifts and guidance. At the 1872 General Conference, the delegates boasted that the "one hundred and twenty-nine laymen here are in the main men of note in their respective localities."[79]

The Reverend Abram Kavanaugh, superintendent of the first hospital in New York, recognized one of the impulses behind the rise of the hospital system: "It is natural," he said, "that the man of commercial instincts should measure our success by the buildings erected, the facilities furnished, and the endowments created.... The philanthropist will ask how many suffering men and women have we restored to their families?" Again and again, hospitals originated through the bequests and gifts of wealthy laity of "commercial instincts" who also considered themselves "philanthropists." The institutions benefited from the small offerings of thousands of humble men and women in the pews of the churches, but those offerings could never have alone resulted in the growth of the Methodist hospital system. The hospitals were built, on the whole, by wealthy laity who saw the buildings as tokens of denominational prestige as well as Christian service.[80]

The Methodists conceived of those hospitals as avenues of service, especially to the needy. They took special pride in what they called "free work" or "gratuitous services" by their physicians, surgeons, and staffs. They referred to the work of their doctors and nurses as "ministries." The hospitals would fulfill the Christian "duty to the sick and suffering of the land, especially to the poor."[81]

The Methodists who founded the hospitals referred to "the example of Wesley" in caring for the sick poor. They saw the hospitals as "deeds of mercy," gifts to humanity. "We have built churches for ourselves and our families," wrote Buckley. "Would it not be well for us soon to build something for all mankind?" And they insisted that Methodist hospitals would receive the poor, not as charity patients but as guests of the Church.[82]

Methodists like to look back on that period of intense construction as a grand epoch of service and sacrifice. It was that, but it was also more. The hospitals may have been built with the poor in mind, but the buildings symbolized the power and affluence of a Methodist tradition that once had suffered condescension from other Protestant groups. Now Methodists constituted a large and affluent membership in a wealthy industrial nation. The proponents of the hospitals warned that the church should not act out of "sectarian ambition," but their reports repeatedly observed that the array of new hospitals could serve as a source of pride and distinction for the church.[83]

It was surely no accident, moreover, that the first public proposal for the construction of hospitals came from James Buckley, who wanted very much to convince the public that Methodism was abreast of the spirit of the age. At the time he wrote his famous editorial, he was engrossed in the controversy over spiritual healing within the denomination. Buckley had argued that the proponents of divine healing were threatening to lead the church into the darkness of superstition and magic. The building of hospitals advertised an alternative piety, attuned to the values of a scientific era, consistent with the spirit of progressive reform, and properly mindful of the professional authority of scientists and doctors. The advocates of the hospitals said explicitly that only through such service to the world could the denomination continue to attract the loyalty of laity in an "ethically minded age."[84]

Like other Protestants, Methodists were aware that the public had long associated hospitals with the Catholic church. On the one hand, the founders of the hospitals noted with admiration and some awe that "the Roman Catholic Church has filled this land with their houses of healing" and that Catholic nuns, especially, seemed willing to take on even the most "heartbreaking" tasks of service to the ill. On the other hand, they observed that Catholic hospitals served as "agencies for disarming suspicion and advancing the ideals of that organization," and they warned that "this work has been left to the Roman Catholics far too long." In an era of intense and sometimes unfriendly competition with Catholicism, Methodists could view their hospitals as an alternative to "the answer of Rome." "Shall Romanism," asked Buckley, "seem to be truer to the benevolent side of the gospel than we are?"[85]

It is useful for several reasons to acknowledge the blurred motives that hid within the grand rhetoric of the denomination. To view the hospitals simply as the incarnations of an ideal of sacrificial service, as after-dinner speakers are wont to view them, runs the risk of idealizing the institutions. An institution analyzed only in ideal categories suffers in the long run, because it escapes painstaking scrutiny by critical minds. A religious tradition that remains sensitive to the nuances of sinfulness will surely remain suspicious of its own motives and institutions.

To idealize the hospitals is to forget that they, like churches and seminaries, stand in need of constant reformation, lest their past unduly control their future. Idealizing rhetoric has a further danger: it overlooks the extent to which hospitalization can be, and often is, an encounter with strangeness, loneliness, and anxiety. Unless we acknowledge that the institutions are human, all too human, we tend to view the anxiety with condescension and impatience. We dismiss it as the petulant ingratitude of patients rather than seeking to make the institution more responsive to human need.

Yet the hospitals served—and still serve—as a commendable, even indispensable, expression of the Methodist tradition, and it is increasingly important in an era of economic stringency to recall the rhetoric, however overblown, that expressed their original purpose. Something of that tradition deserves recall at a time when Methodists are beginning to debate the rationale and plausibility of their commitments to hospitals, which are increasingly viewed as expensive institutions that drain resources needed elsewhere.

In the United States in 1985, Methodists in Kansas debated the proposed sale of a United Methodist hospital to a corporation that would run the institution for profit. The old themes surfaced in new forms. Opponents of the sale argued that "the mission of Christ was to heal the sick and it should be ours," pointing out that health corporations tailor their services to fully insured patients who do not require assistance from governmental programs. They also argued that the sale would be unfair to the region's Catholic hospitals, which did try to serve the poor, by adding to the burden of charity work that the Catholics were carrying. The proponents of the sale replied that the money could be used to pay for other health ministries for the poor, for ethnic minorities, and for rural areas. They argued that the church could no longer afford hospitals and should use its funds for more modest clinics and programs.

The debate was no simple conflict between heartless fiscal conservatives and naive social idealists. It was a complicated discussion about how best to fulfill the mandate of the church, and it ended in an equally complicated compromise. But it probably foreshadows other debates, in which it will be useful to recall both the ambiguity and the idealism of James Buckley's fateful question: "Is it now time that somewhere we built a hospital?"[86]

By the time the debates surfaced, Methodists had moved toward a conception of health quite different from the ones held by their predecessors in the nineteenth century. Rather than thinking of health simply as the absence of impairment, or even as the capacity to enhance physical function, they had begun to conceive of it as the harmonious functioning of a unified person within a community of persons. They became acutely sensitive to the interrelation of body and mind; they thought of persons not as isolated individuals but as complex products of social formation; they viewed illness as a signal of distress within both a physical organism and a social community.

The change resulted primarily from the emerging interest in psychosomatic medicine after the First World War. In England, Leslie Weatherhead began as early as 1922 to push the church to reflect on the ways in which emotional states could create illness. By the 1930s, English Methodists were establishing "healing missions" that combined medical treatment with psychotherapy. In the United States, a Methodist hospital chaplain named Russell Dicks, working alongside the cardiologist Richard Cabot, published in 1936 an influential volume entitled simply *The Art of Ministering to the Sick*. Designed mainly for pastors who visited the sick in hospitals and elsewhere, the book also helped to popularize the awareness that emotions and dispositions could find expression in physical well-being or distress.[87]

Dicks proceeded to publish a series of books and a journal called *Religion and Health* directed both to the sick and to the nurses, doctors, and ministers who cared for them. His theology of health and healing rested on three assumptions, which appeared throughout his writings. First, he believed that the agonies of the soul could create agony in the body. Second, he conceived of God as working "in every case [of illness], struggling to overcome disease and suffering." Indeed, Dicks understood God primarily as a healing power immanent within the natural order, imparting to every creature an inner movement toward health. On occasion he spoke of God as "the great power in ourselves that makes for health," a purposive healing force within each man and woman. Or he wrote of God as "Nature," albeit a nature permeated with purpose and beneficence: "Nature has a way of striking deep within us, of healing things that are broken and giving birth to new things on the earth and in the minds of creatures that pass by." When we understand the working of God in and through nature, he once said, we will speak less of miracle and more of God's constant healing presence. And third, he believed that the sick opened themselves to that presence mainly by the "confession of sins." Growing out of the deepest spiritual needs, confession implied not only a willingness to abandon self-centeredness but also a trust in a reality other than the self. And trust, he thought, was often the precondition of healing.[88]

Dicks's stress on God's immanence within the natural order hardly represented a Methodist consensus. Most Methodists tried to conceive of God as both immanent and transcendent. But even theologians who preferred images of God as a transcendent Sovereign argued increasingly after the Second World War that all healing—even the healing produced through surgery or medication—resulted from an agency that transcended the surgeon, and that the resolution of internal conflict and the forgiveness of sin might well have some bearing not only on the health of the spirit but also on the healing of the body.[89]

In 1942 a Methodist chaplain in America published a book that, more nearly than any other, both summarized and popularized the emerging consensus about health and healing within mainline Methodism. Carroll Wise, who taught pastoral theology for many years at Garrett Biblical Institute in Evanston, Illinois, wrote in his *Religion in Illness and Health* that the "modern approach" to problems of health conceived of the human being as a living unity functioning within an environment, and of religious symbols as powerful realities that could engender growth and integration when rightly understood and produce illness and disintegration when wrongly appropriated. Because the person was a unified organism, he insisted, the minister had to attend not only to the intellectual content of beliefs but to their emotional content as well. When ministers and doctors recognized that religious symbols revealed a disposition and orientation of a unified self, they would gain a fresh insight into both religion and health.[90]

Wise was interested in the function of religious symbols, but he did not make the simplistic claim that men and women should be religious for the sake of being healthy. Nor did he argue that religious symbols merely reflected psychological states. He contended that the symbols could uncover truths about reality that were as "inescapable as the law of gravitation." God could not be viewed merely as an ideal, useful for psychological well-being. The Christian use of the term *God* pointed rather to an inescapable reality, and the language with which Christians spoke of God served as rules for a "continuous reorientation of life" toward that reality. Because the reorientation involved unified persons in their wholeness, it invariably had a crucial bearing on their health and well-being.[91]

Similar views came to characterize the discussions of the Methodist Society for Medical and Pastoral Practice in England. Erastus Evans warned that religious faith offered no set of manipulable techniques to make the work of physicians easier; yet it remained true, he added, that spiritual disturbance affected the whole of a person's life. William Strawson emphasized that theologians could not "explain the facts of disease and the technique of cure in terms of divine providence and human activity"; but the theologian, he said, did have to assert that "the secret of any effective healing is co-operation with the divine forces of healing" through a disposition of trust and confidence.[92]

Implicit—and often explicit—in the new understandings of health and healing was a depiction of the person as an organism seeking integration or fulfillment or wholeness. The vocabulary revealed the extent of the theologians' debt to the psychologists and practitioners of psychosomatic medicine. Yet the language of "integration" and "fulfillment" had an obvious affinity with an older Wesleyan vocabulary that had spoken of the Christian life as a journey, a development from prevenient grace to entire sanctification. And the metaphor of wholeness clearly suggested an older metaphor of holiness.

Because of its debt to pietism and its revivalistic fervor, Methodism had always attended carefully to the interior growth of the soul, and Wesley had entertained his notions of health and healing within a broader understanding of spiritual development. It was surely no surprise, then, that Wesley's heirs in the twentieth century found themselves attracted to depictions of health that emphasized the relation between the well-being of the body and the integrated growth of the whole person.

The expansive conception of health that has marked much Methodist activity within the past half-century represents an appropriate sensitivity to the complexity of the concepts of health and well-being. But it also conceals a hidden danger: that health and well-being will be conceived as one and the same. When that happens, the ethical and religious dimensions of human existence, complex beyond description, collapse into the one dimension of health, forcing physicians who make medical judgments to assume "responsibility for the full range of human moral considerations."[93] Physicians are not quite ready to bear that burden. Human well-being is a complicated matter that requires serious ethical and religious reflection as well as serious medical inquiry.

Methodists also require an occasional salutary warning that a preoccupation with growth and development, especially when recast in a modern vocabulary of fulfillment and self-realization, can degenerate easily into a self-preoccupation that serves its own ends, including the ends of bodily health and psychological well-being. When that happens, piety becomes an instrumental pietism, faith becomes a technique, and health becomes the highest good rather than merely a means to a higher good.

But a piety of sanctification, of holiness, or of wholeness, if you will, need not lead to a legalism of the spirit or an idolatry of the heart. At its best, the piety of sanctification does not conform reality to the self; it rather forms the self by directing it outside itself. When growth, whether spiritual or psychological, becomes an end consciously sought, the end proves elusive, for a self-arranged growth remains within the narrow boundaries of the self that arranges it. But when the self is drawn outside itself, when the journey focuses the gaze on the truth rather than on the traveler who seeks the truth, then the truth can indeed make one whole. And when that wholeness brings health and healing, the traveler will be grateful for the gift.

# Part II

# VALLEYS OF THE SHADOW

# ·3·

# Suffering

A friend of Wesley named Alexander Knox once wrote him during an illness and told him that he was prepared to accept suffering because he had "no right" to expect the continuance of his health. In his return letter, Wesley acknowledged that his friend had no right to expect the cessation of suffering as a claim on God's justice. It was true, Wesley said, that Knox did not "merit it at [God's] hands." But Wesley then dissented from his friend's judgment. God's justice, he said, is not the measure whereby God invariably dealt with the creature. "Does He give us no more blessings than we deserve? Does He treat us in all things according to His justice? Not so: but mercy rejoices over judgment. Therefore expect from him not what you deserve, but what you want—health of soul and health of body." The resigned acceptance of suffering was no necessary duty.[1]

A friend of Wesley named Mary Bishop once informed him, with some distress, about her own suffering. In subsequent letters to her, Wesley seemed to give quite a different account of suffering and resignation to it. He told her that he had often found pain and sickness to be of considerable benefit to the spirit. "It is an admirable help against levity, as well as against foolish desires; and nothing more directly tends to teach us that great lesson, to write upon our heart, 'not as I will, but as thou wilt.'" Suffering, he told her later, was one of the "grand means which God employs" to draw the heart from worldliness to piety.[2]

In the not so subtle contrast between the letter to Knox and those to Bishop, Wesley elaborated a theological conundrum which would occupy the Methodist tradition for two centuries. Was suffering a curse or a gift? An enemy or a friend in disguise? Was it to be fought or accepted? Did it embody God's purposes or did it contradict God's merciful intention for the creature? Wesley thought that he could answer these questions. Later

Methodists were not always certain that they could. Wesley's own answers can be best understood, and the contrasts in the letters made intelligible, through his metaphor of the Christian journey.

## HOLINESS AND HAPPINESS

One can summarize Wesley's answers with a simple formulation: suffering is not the purpose of the journey, but suffering need not be merely a barrier along the way. The two sides of the formulation require a balanced emphasis. Wesley did not believe that men and women were simply to endure earthly existence or think of it as a salutary course of suffering to prepare the soul for another world. Yet suffering for Wesley did not negate happiness. It could serve, he thought, as the avenue to a happiness beyond the happiness that the soul originally envisioned.

The historical theologian Albert Outler, after spending a lifetime studying Wesley's works, finally concluded that "this man was a *eudaemonist*, convinced and consistent all his life. All his emphases on duty and discipline are auxiliary to his main concern for human *happiness*." Far from romanticizing suffering or viewing it as the normal expectation for a fallen world, Wesley interpreted the whole Christian story of fall and redemption as an epic with happiness as a central theme. It is true, he said, that pain and suffering followed the Fall, but he added that God could have permitted a fall only with the intention of ultimately increasing human happiness by providing men and women with a deeper vision of the divine life as redemptive and reconciling. Far from thinking that holiness precluded happiness, Wesley preached that only the holy were truly happy, and that the truly unhappy were also unholy, that is, unable truly to love.[3]

Suffering, then, was not to be sought but to be overcome. Wesley's preoccupation with health and medicine grew out of his belief that the law of love drew the Christian into a constant battle against suffering. His dispensaries and his medical tracts issued from the same sensibility that produced his polemic against slavery, his care for the poor, his criticism of prostitution (which he entitled, characteristically, "A Word to an Unhappy Woman"), his dismay at alcoholism, his worries about hunger in England, and his creation of schools and orphanages. The primary task when faced with suffering was to overcome it, for suffering was an enemy, not a friend.

Yet even the enemy could serve as a guide. So intense was Wesley's devotion to happiness that he could not abandon the hope that even the enemy was a friend in disguise. He acknowledged that human nature shrank from pain, and he thought it blameless in doing so. The Christian had every right to pray for release from pain: "If it be possible, let this cup pass from me" (Matthew 26:39a). Even so, Wesley thought that the Christian had also the duty of adding a second prayer: "Nevertheless, not as I will, but as Thou wilt" (Matthew 26:39b). He had no hesitance in calling for resignation to suffering, because he conceived of afflictions as blessings through which God conveyed gracious benefits. Sickness and pain could bring conversion and assurance and holiness. "You have accordingly found pain, sickness, bodily weakness to be real goods," he wrote to a friend, "as bringing you nearer and nearer to the fountain of all happiness and holiness."[4]

His confidence in the purposefulness of pain reflected a conviction that pain could be borne. Christians did not fear pain, he wrote, for they knew that it would never be sent unless for their own real advantage and that their strength would be "proportioned to it, as it always has been in times past." He taught that the appropriate response to suffering was always "patience," a disposition of creatures who took suffering seriously, never dismissing it simply as an accident or a chance occurrence, but also never permitting it to affect them overmuch, to overpower and dissolve them. Patience was not what Wesley thought of as "Stoical insensibility." He thought that Christians could hurt and mourn; they could acknowledge pain as painful, without trying to deny the hurt or to disguise the hope that it might pass away. Patience was the faith that pain bore a meaning beyond itself, that it created a pathway to holiness and hence, mysteriously, to happiness.[5]

Wesley's father once lay in pain for seven months. On one occasion Wesley asked him: "Sir, are you in pain now?" His father answered: "God does indeed chasten me with pain; yea, all my bones with strong pain. But I thank him for all; I bless him for all; I love him for all." Wesley considered the answer to be exemplary, and it inevitably made its way into his sermons. It provided for him a concrete illustration of his faith that suffering could form holiness, and holiness could engender happiness, and happiness could fulfill the intention of the creator for the creation.[6]

## SUFFERING AND MADNESS

The topics of insanity, emotional pain, and madness are part of Wesley's larger conception of suffering. He discussed those topics frequently, in part because he constantly had to counter charges that his own revivalist activities drove people mad. He acknowledged that when other denominations of Christians thought about Methodists, their first thought was that "much religion hath made them mad." And he agreed that certain forms of religious "enthusiasm" could properly be construed as a species of madness, arising from fantasies of divine inspiration. He agreed even that "touches of extravagance, bordering on madness," could arise from a true conviction of sin produced by a true religious insight. But on the whole he considered it silliness when zealous Christians were "branded with the names of madmen and enthusiasts." What the world often accounted madness, he said, was simply an appropriate contempt for merely temporal goods.[7]

True madness, he thought, was a complicated form of suffering, caused by a complex variety of physical and spiritual agencies. The suffering of madness resulted often from the sickness of the body. "Let but the blood move irregularly in the brain, and all regular thinking is at an end. Raging madness ensues; and then farewell to all evenness of thought." Even lesser forms of mental suffering could have their origin in bodily disorders. It seemed sometimes to Wesley that the soul sympathized with the body, so that acute disease and violent pain, or even chronic diseases with few painful symptoms, lured the soul into a debilitating "heaviness."[8]

Other nervous disorders might result from irregular passions. Wesley believed that inordinate passions could damage the nerves. Even violent joy, though it raised the spirits for a time, tended afterward to sink them into depression. "And every one knows," he said, "what an influence fear has upon our whole frame." If mental passions could leave their imprint even on the mysterious dreams of the night, they could surely produce other changes in human consciousness, however little we might understand them.[9]

Still other instances of mental suffering, though, resulted from the agency of demonic powers. Wesley once asked an "experienced physician," eminent for curing madness, if he had any reason to believe that "most lunatics are demoniacs." The physician gave Wesley the answer he wanted to hear: "Sir, I have been often inclined to think, that most lunatics are demoniacs. Nor is there any weight in that objection, that they are frequently cured by medicine: for so might any other disease, occasioned by an evil spirit, if God did not suffer him to repeat the stroke, by which the disease is occasioned." Satan surely knew enough about human physiology, Wesley thought, to act upon "those parts in the animal machine which are more immediately subservient to thinking" and thereby "raise a thousand perceptions and emotions in the mind, so far as God is pleased to permit."[10]

Wesley knew that it was no longer fashionable among the intellectuals of Europe to attribute mental illness to satanic agency. He often betrayed the annoyance and defensiveness of the true believer who finds conviction met by ridicule. But it was precisely his continued attachment to an unfashionable conviction that permitted Wesley to recognize the flaw in more fashionable explanations of mental illness. The "wise men" explain madness by appealing to theories about the nerves, he complained. But they knew nothing about the nerves, so that what seemed to be an explanation turned out to be a circular definition: mental illness, about which little was known, had its origins in the nerves, about which nothing certain was known. Hence one unknown became an explanation for another unknown. Wesley preferred to talk about demons and spirits. Recent generations of Methodists have, on the whole, found Wesley's assertions about the demonic etiology of mental illness to be a curious fragment of their distant past. But the accidental insight about clinical language needs to be remembered, for circular explanations did not cease in the eighteenth century.[11]

He also recognized, as his successors have recognized, that mental disorders could on occasion have their ground in a genuine spiritual malaise, an absence of any sense of meaning. Nervous disorders, he said, particularly the disorders that physicians could not explain, sometimes masked a deeper sickness of the spirit, an elusive, almost unconscious sense of the absence of meaning. They could have their source in a "dull consciousness of the want of God, and the unsatisfactoriness of every thing here below." Or they could result from genuine guilt, from a "conviction of sin" that arose from the fact of having lived sinfully and without love.[12]

The world was full, then, of madness, of every kind and intensity—the madness of chemical imbalance, the madness of emotional disarray, the madness of demonic malice, and the madness of spiritual malaise. And that listing was not exhaustive. Wesley considered even anger to be a form of madness. He recognized other forms stemming from diet, alcoholism, or spiritual and physical lassitude.[13]

Whatever the form of madness, it represented suffering, and Wesley considered it the Christian's duty to struggle against it. It is true that some of his own prescriptions now seem quaint. In his *Primitive Physick* he suggested treating lunacy by rubbing the head with a mixture of vinegar and ground ivy leaves, or swallowing an ounce of distilled vinegar each day, or applying electricity. For "raging madness," he suggested applying wet packs or pouring a steady stream of water on the head, or trying a diet solely of apples or of bread and milk. But he recognized the need for some kind of medical treatment, even when the origin of the disease seemed to be demonic: "We are, even in that weakness, to use natural means, just as if it was owing to natural causes."[14]

He recognized also that the treatment could be as painful as the disease and that the methods of treatment required constant criticism and reassessment. Confinement in Bethlehem Hospital—the notorious "Bedlam"—could itself drive a person mad, he said. And he criticized the common practice of physically beating the insane. Some forms of treatment, in short, bore little effect and produced precisely the unhappiness that medical treatment was designed to alleviate. The aim of treatment was the restoration of happiness. Mental sufferings required care because they were "enemies to the joy of faith." In the restoring of joy, the physician had the duty not to impose unnecessarily another form of joylessness.[15]

Just as he had refused to deny the reality of physical sufferings, Wesley refused to treat mental disorders simply by urging the sufferer to take heart and be faithful. He recognized, for one thing, that facile attempts to assert the curative power of "faith"—even of a genuine faithfulness—often ran up against the sheer reality of natural suffering: "Faith does not overturn the course of nature," he said. "Natural causes still produce natural effects." Faith no more hindered "the sinking of the spirits (as it is called) in an hysteric illness, than the rising of the pulse in a fever." He did not make the error that became common among many of his successors; he did not treat faith as a psychologically beneficial means of therapy. He may in his youth have veered too near the boundaries of a theological legalism, but he did not in his maturity fall into the therapeutic legalism which confused religious faith with positive thinking.[16]

Despite Wesley's interest in the theme of madness, the Methodist tradition has produced no extensive body of writing and reflection about mental illness. The Methodist churches and hospitals have, however, continued the effort to minister to the mentally ill. As early as 1868, a Methodist General Conference in America approved the appointment of chaplains to institutions for persons suffering from mental illness. The church's interest in mental health intensified after the inauguration in 1909 of the mental hygiene movement in America and Europe. Both clergy and laity gave their support to the movement's efforts to reform mediocre hospitals and promote mental health in local communities. In the 1920s, some of the clergy who shared those interests in mental health entered programs in clinical pastoral education, which exposed theological students to the suffering of persons who were mentally ill.

Such exposure to clinical training led Carroll Wise, Methodist chaplain at the Worcester State Hospital in Massachusetts, eventually to conclude that "mental hospital experience leads to a broadening and deepening of one's views on life, health, and religion." He therefore joined others in looking afresh at the function of religious symbols in the creation or destruction of mental stability. In arguing that questions of meaning and value can "in specific ways affect the health of the individual," Wise urged the churches to recover the Wesleyan interest in the suffering of the mentally ill.[17]

A small but active group of Methodist clergy and laity began during the 1940s to explore the ways in which the churches themselves could diminish the pain of emotional suffering, whether by joining with organizations devoted to the reform of public hospitals or by sponsoring local fellowships, organizations, and gatherings which could promote mental health. Paul Maves of Drew University argued that by recovering Wesley's awareness of the healing potential of small, intimate groups, the churches could "discharge more adequately their responsibility for helping persons . . . maintain mental and emotional equilibrium."[18]

In 1964 Methodists in the United States added to their Social Creed a new section on mental health and medical care. They supported both governmental and private research in public health, and called for adequate facilities and staffs to aid the emotionally ill and the mentally retarded "of every community."[19] The real struggle to sustain mental health, however, has more often occurred in local congregations, where small groups provide support for their members. Occasionally, those congregations have developed impressive programs of outreach to other sufferers.

As one example, consider the resolve of the Metropolitan United Methodist Church in Detroit to draw mentally retarded adults into its life and activities. Its pastor, William Quick, appealed to other congregations "to become aware of retarded persons and to do something to make them a part of a loving Christian fellowship."

> In an age when most folk walk on the other side of the street to avoid the mentally retarded adult, these "special children" of God have found what it really means to be accepted within the Christian fellowship. . . . Our entire church has become conscious of a world of persons who have, for the most part, been "hidden away" from the rest of us. Their presence has sensitized the church to the reality that persons of limited possibilities are indeed inheritors of God's grace.[20]

In such ways have Methodists carried forward Wesley's conviction that mental illness represented a form of suffering against which the Christian should struggle.

## HOLINESS AGAINST HAPPINESS

Wesley persisted in thinking about suffering in a larger context of happiness and holiness. His theology sometimes ran the risk of denying the reality of suffering by treating it simply as a blessing in disguise, for to view suffering as a disguised blessing is to view it as something other than suffering and hence to underestimate its power. But more often his language about happiness and holiness provided a way to recognize the reality of suffering while refusing to concede that a suffering which was real must therefore be utterly without meaning.

To understand the insight in Wesley's coupling of suffering with the themes of happiness and holiness, one must recall that in his theology the "way of salvation," the Christian journey, was a way of love. In linking pain to happiness and holiness, Wesley was trying to affirm that suffering could deepen the life of love. By that he meant that love responded to the suffering of others, and it did so by taking that suffering seriously.

He also meant that suffering can engender the capacity to love. He did not say that it *must* engender that capacity. He did not think of suffering in terms of the ethical demands that it imposed. But he recognized that suffering could, in fact, deepen within the sufferer the ability to love other sufferers, as well as to love the God who, in the Son, also suffered. The sufferer could learn to love, and the love born of suffering could bear a meaning, even a happiness and joy, within its depths.

That idea coincided with another theme in his theology, which would often reappear in the Wesleyan tradition: that suffering became meaningful for the Christian insofar as it came to represent for the sufferer a participation in the sufferings of Christ. Wesley tended to speak often of Christ as the "pattern" of the Christian life. To suffer was to assume one's place within the form of life shaped by the pattern of the Christ on the cross. Wesley sought always to have "the mind that was in Christ"; he believed that suffering could help to form the mind of Christ within the Christian by intensifying the depth of both happiness and holiness.[21]

Within a few years of Wesley's death in 1791, his rhetorical linkage between happiness and holiness began to fade into the background of Methodist teaching. Increasingly, Methodists would speak as if deep holiness stood in contrast to shallow happiness, and once the separation of holiness and happiness became established, the understanding of suffering also shifted subtly.

The shift was visible in the *Theological Institutes* written by Richard Watson, the first English systematizer of Wesleyan thought. Writing for what was becoming a denomination of shopkeepers and greengrocers, Watson wanted to demonstrate the reasonableness and responsibility of Methodism within a culture that still thought of Wesleyans as sectarian fanatics. Like other conventional theologians of his era, Watson talked about the evidences of Christianity and the ethical duties of Christians. He tended therefore to locate his discussions of suffering within the section of his theology devoted to "the morals of Christianity." His central theme was that submission to God's will was one of the "duties we owe to God." The Christian virtue of trust entailed a resignation to God's will and a courageous acceptance of suffering. The virtue of trust elevated the soul "above all cowardly shrinking from difficulty, suffering, pain, and death." The virtue of resignation and the hope of heaven reconciled the Christian to the pain of bodily sufferings. Watson found meaning in suffering by shifting the focus from happiness (and hence from the way in which suffering could nurture the capacity to love) to duty (and hence to the way in which suffering could embody the virtue of obedience).[22]

When the Asiatic cholera appeared in England in 1831, the Methodists of London called for fasting and humiliation. They also asked Watson to address them. He began by sharing further bad news: "I am sorry to inform you," he said, "that the news from the north, received today, is unfavourable. Five more cases of cholera have occurred; and three of them have been fatal." He then proceeded to preach from the book of 2 Samuel, reminding his listeners that God had also sent a pestilence upon Israel. As the prophets had called for Israel to repent, so Watson called for his listeners to confess their sins, and his concluding prayer listed "with minuteness and particularity" the "sins of individuals, of the church, and of the nation." Watson assured his congregation that "all things shall work together for good to them that love [the Lord]," but he also urged them to assume the responsibility for the suffering and to undertake the Christian duty of confession.[23]

The Methodist theologians of the early nineteenth century often assumed the task of justifying the ways of God. They tried to show that suffering was meaningful and that God was therefore blameless. The American theologian Albert Taylor Bledsoe illustrated a common pattern. In a little book entitled *Theodicy*, published in 1854, he argued that suffering resulted from sinfulness, and that its meaning was to be found in its capacity to form holiness. The existence of sin and evil could be reconciled with the power and goodness of God, he thought, only if the grand aim and design of God's moral government was the production of the greatest possible amount of moral good. Such a design presupposed the existence of temptation, the freedom to sin, and the possibility of misery, all being necessary to the attainment of virtue. Moral character, not happiness, was the goal of human existence, and suffering was necessary for the formation of moral character.[24]

The themes of resignation, duty, and character became the staples of Wesleyan devotional writing on the theme of suffering throughout the early nineteenth century. Like other Christians in England and America, Wesleyans created a veritable "cult of frailty," in which physical suffering and resignation to it became marks of piety. In the devotional guidebooks for the sick and bereaved that became popular in the 1830s, suffering was the occasion to learn patient submission, to yield all attachments to temporal goods, to testify to God's goodness, and to seek a future happiness in another world.

The same themes had appeared in Wesley's sermons, but by placing them within a larger vision of holiness and happiness, and by defining both happiness and holiness as the deepening of the capacity for love, Wesley had described a religious possibility more than he had prescribed an ethical duty intended for the cultivation of moral character. The early nineteenth-century theologians placed the accent on duty.[25]

By the late nineteenth century, the Methodist systematic theologian at Garrett Biblical Institute, Miner Raymond, was arguing that one could understand suffering within God's moral government only by recognizing that "holiness, and not happiness, is the true and supreme end of being." For Raymond, love had become not so much a gift as an "obligation," and happiness not the fulfillment of love but an alternative to it. Suffering was a means to an end, and the end was something other than Wesley's "happiness."[26]

There were other perspectives on suffering in the nineteenth century, especially among the black Methodists who endured chattel slavery in America. When Richard Allen of the African Methodist Episcopal Church wrote of suffering, he included the standard topics, but for him the significant point was that Jesus had never omitted the opportunity of doing good to the bodies of the multitudes who came to him "laboring under sickness and disorders." The lesson was that Christians were to go and do likewise. When Daniel Payne of the African Methodist Episcopal Church wrote of suffering, he, too, included the standard themes, but for him the central point was that the Christian was to plead the cause of the oppressed, not simply from sympathy toward the suffering, but because the living God had commanded it.[27]

In their accent on the duties of love to the suffering, the black theologians pointed the way toward the Methodist social gospel of the late nineteenth century. Both in England and in America, Wesleyan theologians began to embrace a vision of suffering as a corporate reality which could be opposed only through corporate effort. To address the physical suffering of the poor, wrote Hugh Price Hughes in London, the Christian had to "elect vestry-men who would close unsanitary dwellings." Doing so, he added, embodied the heart of the Wesleyan tradition: "When John Wesley looked forth on Christendom . . . God inspired him with love for the neglected masses. That was the secret of the triumph of early Methodism."[28]

The theologians of a social Methodism believed that the task of love was to labor on behalf of the earth's miserably unhappy. One was to concentrate one's attention on the miseries that could be overcome, not on metaphysical quandaries that defied resolution. "Disease," wrote Hughes, "is an avoidable and a removable evil." He considered it intolerable that a Christian nation—for he thought of England as a Christian nation—would permit avoidable evils to continue. The problem of suffering required not resignation but active struggle. The possibility implicit in suffering was not so much the deepening of holiness as it was the relief of pain. Suffering was no friend in disguise; suffering was the enemy, relentless and merciless.[29]

Christians opposed suffering because they understood human reality from the standpoint of a suffering divine reality. Hughes appealed to the depiction of a suffering Christ on a cross. Christ's suffering, he said, was deep and intense; he underwent both physical misery and utter separation from God, all in order to identify himself fully with us. Hence those who followed in the way of the Christ had no real choice but to identify themselves with Jesus as he had identified himself with the misery of humanity. And just as his identification of himself with us took the form of his placing himself at our service, so our identification of ourselves with him required that we place ourselves at his service. For a nineteenth-century social Methodist, the meaning of that requirement seemed clear; the service of Christ meant, above all, the life of active love. "We are to love each other even as Christ loves us." In loving each other, we devote ourselves to relieving the other's pain.[30]

In the course of Methodist history in the nineteenth century, therefore, the older Wesleyan conjunction of happiness and holiness fell apart, with the result that for a while Methodist understandings of suffering moved in two different directions. The Methodist theologians who maintained a piety of resignation tended to counterpose happiness and holiness, and to view suffering as a means of holiness, a friend in disguise. For them, love within suffering took the form of resignation to the will of God. The resignation embodied confidence that a fuller happiness awaited in a future life free of all suffering and pain. "Jesus, lover of my soul, / Let me to thy bosom fly, / While the nearer waters roll, / While the tempest still is high: / Hide me, O my Savior, hide / Till the storm of life is past; / Safe into the haven guide; / O receive my soul at last."³¹

The Methodist theologians who advocated a piety of service tended also to counterpose happiness and holiness, not explicitly, but by attending single-mindedly to the task of seeking a measure of happiness for the miserable. They viewed suffering as a barrier to happiness, not as a friend in disguise. For them, love within suffering took the form of service to the other as an expression of service to God. And the service occurred not only in a distant future but also in the effort to create the loving and beloved community here and now. "To serve the present age, / my calling to fulfill; / O may it all my powers engage / To do my Master's will."³²

Each of the Wesleyan options—the piety of inwardness and the piety of service—harbored a risk. On the one side, the theologians of resignation seemed so intent on discovering the usefulness of suffering that they lost sight of its sheer misery. And by speaking of resignation to suffering as a duty, thereby interpreting it as an ethical category, they fell into theological disarray. The endurance of suffering became an achievement of the will; failure to achieve it called for reproof and blame. By implication, the Christian life became a series of tests and trials to be overcome for the sake of proving one's own worthiness. It is hard to deny that the theologians of resignation blurred the Christian understanding of life as a gift to be received with thankfulness. It is hard to interpret suffering as a duty without interpreting complaint as ethical failure.

And yet, before we too harshly judge the theology of resignation, it is well for us to remember that there are times when resignation to inevitable suffering, intractable and unavoidable suffering, may be a realistic choice. When rebellion against suffering only intensifies the pain, especially when it only intensifies the pain of the sufferer's beloved, it would seem perverse to deplore resignation as somehow "bad." The mistake of these theologians was that they tended to make resignation an ethical obligation and to respond with blame when the obligation seemed unfulfilled. But it must be granted that, in some moments, resignation can represent an appropriate insight into the intractability and evil of suffering.

On the other side, the theologians of service seemed so intent on overcoming avoidable sufferings that they neglected to reflect on the unavoidable ones. They recognized love's opposition to needless suffering, and they did not impose on the sufferer the duty of resignation. But they had little to say about inexorable suffering—the suffering that would remain despite the best intentions of the most well-meaning community. Their sense of the tragic appeared diminished or incomplete. As men and women living with others each day, they shared fully in the sufferings of friends and strangers. The pioneers of the social gospel seem, in retrospect, to have been an extraordinarily sensitive and caring group of people. But as theologians, they felt more comfortable dealing with manageable sufferings than with intransigent and inevitable suffering.

But before we judge the theologians of service as being superficial and excessively optimistic, it is well to remember that they faithfully represented for their era the Wesleyan insight that we are not here to suffer. In choosing to struggle against sufferings that seemed vulnerable to conquest, they assumed no small task, for those sufferings resisted tenaciously. Our own era, deeply impressed by the tragic ironies of suffering and by its intractability, can easily use the charge of superficiality as an excuse for our own refusal to battle against manageable sufferings that we could possibly overcome.

One might next expect a synthesis combining the best of both traditions. But such a synthesis would be artificial: to view both resignation and resistance, in their nineteenth-century forms, as appropriate responses to suffering is to entertain a contradiction. Yet Methodists have tried to move beyond the impasse, not by synthesizing nineteenth-century conflicts but by seeking older patterns of thought, present both in the eighteenth century and in the first.

## HOLINESS AND HAPPINESS REVISITED

Wesley tried to understand suffering by conjoining the themes of happiness and holiness. At first glance, the conjunction seems curious. On later reflection, it can seem almost perverse. Who can observe the intensity of suffering in a hospital, or the loving pain of parents who cherish a retarded child, or the misery of a schizophrenic teenager, and speak still of holiness and happiness? Especially in an era that links the image of happiness with the absence of suffering—indeed, that distinguishes only with great difficulty between happiness and pleasure—who can dare even to utter the word in the presence of horrible pain?

Who knows, for that matter, how to define, let alone understand, either happiness or holiness? A cursory look at the history of Christianity, even of Wesleyan Christianity, reveals the shifting conceptions of the holy. And as for happiness, the term can seem purely formal and empty. The nineteenth-century Methodist theologian Borden Bowne delighted in exhibiting the ambiguities hidden in the word *happiness*. Of course it is right, he said, to seek happiness. Even ascetics who scorn happiness seek a higher well-being that might appropriately be designated as a higher "happiness." But what is happiness? "The difficulty with eudaemonism is not that it is false," he said, "but that it is a barren truism." The term is so vague as to furnish no guidance whatever for our actions and no insight into our suffering.[33]

The problem seemed inconsequential to Wesley, however, and it serves us well to ask why. It is at least possible that the larger pattern of affirmations and denials in the Wesleyan vision made it seem plausible, at least in the eighteenth century, to engage the dilemmas of suffering by talking of happiness and holiness. By locating the language of happiness and holiness within a broader context of theological affirmations, one finds that both terms function together in ways that are neither empty nor insensitive. They provided guideposts within a journey that was no aimless wandering, and the larger journey set the meaning of the guideposts along the way.

The journey, we recall, was the "way of salvation," which for Wesley meant the way of love. Both happiness and holiness functioned in Wesleyan theology as pointers designating something about love. Wesley conceived of holiness as an ability (not simply a capacity) to love, and as the expression of that ability in loving dispositions. Though he never, to my knowledge, offered a precise definition of happiness, he clearly understood it to be an awareness that issued from the ability to attend lovingly to a reality other than oneself. Hence the highest happiness was to be found in a love for God, an enrapt devotion that drew our attention from ourselves and directed it outside ourselves. The result of that attentiveness to other realities was the absence of self-consciousness and the anxiety that accompanies self-consciousness.

Both holiness and happiness, therefore, were modes of the same reality: love. Holiness was the ability to love; happiness was the fulfillment of love. It was fulfillment as the sheer enjoyment of love, the enjoyment of the beloved and the enjoyment that comes from being able to accept and receive love. The happiness of love was the self-transcendence of love, which pointed always beyond itself, though it did so within a relationship of mutuality that permitted it to rejoice also in receiving the love of the other, be it the love of God or of other persons. Surely, then, it makes sense to conjoin the themes of suffering and love. Indeed, that conjunction might make more sense than any other.

When one speaks of love and happiness from within a Methodist setting, one echoes Wesley's conviction that we are not here to suffer. When surgeons in the nineteenth century began to use anesthetics to deaden the pain of surgical operations, other surgeons objected, sometimes on the theological grounds that pain had been a necessary part of the human condition ever since the Fall. Doubtless some of those pious proponents of suffering were Methodists. But they surely had wandered beyond the boundaries of their own heritage, for Wesley was certain that happiness, not pain, was the purpose of the human journey. Despite his conviction that God could and did use suffering to turn the wayward heart, Wesley denied that suffering could appropriately be described as God's intention for the creation, even for the fallen creation.[34]

When one speaks of love and holiness from within a Methodist setting, one echoes Wesley's conviction that suffering need not be utterly meaningless. To be sure, Wesley was far more explicit about its possible meanings than most of his twentieth-century heirs would venture to be. But even the Methodists of a chastened twentieth century have been willing to join in the minimal assertion that suffering need not be utterly meaningless. And like Wesley, they have often been inclined to discover its meaning in the possibilities of love that it can foster.

One treads softly in making such an assertion, lest one return to the ethical legalism of the nineteenth-century theologians of inwardness. It does not seem useful to insist that love is a duty of the sufferer, as those theologians insisted on the duty of resignation. Yet the remark that suffering can foster love seems both an accurate observation and a useful insight, however simple and commonplace. One need not say that the fostering of love is the "purpose" of suffering in order to recognize the possibility, the sheer possibility, that suffering can enhance and deepen the ability to love other sufferers. And insofar as it deepens the ability to love, suffering is not entirely without meaning. The Wesleyan notion of happiness serves as a warning against facile assertions about the "purpose" of suffering. The Wesleyan notion of holiness serves as a warning against premature assertions about the "purposelessness" of suffering.

Methodist theologians, like other theologians, have often attempted to address the mystery of suffering by providing explanations. John Wesley in the eighteenth century assumed that suffering was an ingredient within a redemptive order that aimed at the happiness of the creature. Albert Taylor Bledsoe in the nineteenth century explained that suffering was intended for the strengthening of moral character. Edgar Sheffield Brightman in the twentieth concluded that the reality of suffering required the theologian to assert the finitude of God. Working within the philosophical tradition of personalism at Boston University, Brightman argued that a truly personal God, truly good and truly related to the created order, obviously was a God who struggled against evil without in every instance overcoming it. Indeed, the intractability of suffering suggested that even God struggled with a reality that remained a resistant given in the divine experience.[35]

Brightman's reflections about the finitude of God represented a minority voice within the tradition, but similar speculative accounts have had widespread currency in twentieth-century Methodism. Leslie Weatherhead's brief treatise on *The Will of God*, published in 1944 in England in the midst of war, has remained a familiar text in congregational study groups attempting to understand suffering. Weatherhead wrote the pamphlet to discourage the assumption, which he had repeatedly encountered, that the death of a child or the suffering of a friend could be considered the "will of God." The assumption, he thought, reflected a confusion.

He hoped to resolve the confusion by distinguishing God's intentional, circumstantial, and ultimate will. The intentional will of God, he argued, embodied the ideal divine plan for humanity: mutuality and happiness. God did not will suffering. But God created men and women as free creatures, and their freedom implied an ability to create suffering. Hence the need to talk of God's circumstantial will. When human freedom frustrated God's intentional will, God did not remove the freedom. Instead, God worked within the suffering, and only in that sense could the suffering be attributed to the will of God. God's intention, for instance, was that the men and women of the first century would have understood and received the message of Jesus and realized his kingdom. They chose, instead, to crucify him. In those circumstances, the cross and its suffering were God's will. But God willed the cross only because the abuse of freedom made it necessary. And the cross then became a means by which God realized the ideal purposes originally envisioned in the divine plan. In that sense, the cross could be described as God's ultimate will, ultimate because it represented the final realization of the divine purposes.[36]

The divine will, then, operated within restrictions. God as redeemer honored the natural regularities established by God as creator. God did not set aside the natural laws that governed the created order. Hence the law of gravity created suffering for the child who fell from a ladder. God did not will the pain, but God also did not set aside the physiological laws of pain that governed bodily existence. God as redeemer, moreover, honored the moral regularities established by God as creator. God did not set aside the moral freedom that marked the human order. Hence the weapons of war created suffering for the soldier who died in battle. God did not will the death, but God also did not set aside the moral freedom that permitted wars to occur. Hence the pain might be called God's circumstantial will. But God's intentional will was a will for human happiness, not human suffering, and God's ultimate will would ensure that the original intention would somehow be realized. God would reach at last the ultimate goal, and nothing of value would be finally lost.[37]

Weatherhead's distinctions permitted him to argue that the pain and suffering of sickness could not be interpreted as the result of God's intention. The doctors and nurses who labored to overcome the suffering were not somehow violating the divine will. But because God could use a cross, God could also use pain and suffering to achieve an ultimate good, and one could therefore speak of a "will of God" within the circumstances of sickness. God's will within the conditions of disease was that the sufferer bear the suffering in such a way as both to enrich the community of sufferers and to enhance the sufferer's own capacity to love.[38]

As a piece of metaphysical explanation, Weatherhead's treatise clearly failed. He acknowledged as much. He had no way of explaining why the will of the Creator permitted germs and malignant cells. He assumed that the misuse of human freedom explained virtually every human ill, but he recognized the existence of ills that could not be traced to moral flaws. Yet despite its metaphysical incompleteness, Weatherhead's argument reflected the continuing themes of holiness and happiness within the Wesleyan tradition. Like Wesley, he insisted that suffering was not the divine purpose. Like Wesley, he insisted that suffering need not be meaningless. Like Wesley, he affirmed that suffering had a meaning beyond the meanings we can imagine.

Because metaphysical explanations of suffering and evil have invariably proven to be inadequate, most Methodist theologians have chosen another way of understanding theologically the mystery of suffering. They have acknowledged its resistance to rational explanation, but they have not therefore chosen to remain silent. Instead, they have observed that the New Testament speaks less about the will of a powerful and distant deity than about the suffering of the man Jesus in whom God dwelt. They have emphasized that the ancient creeds speak less about God's will than about God's incarnation within a suffering humanity as one who also suffered. They have written less about God's ideal plan than about the proclamation of the New Testament that a cross and a resurrection shape the Christian depiction of our common life together. To speak in this manner is not to provide satisfactory metaphysical explanations. It is simply to interpret our sufferings by locating them within the narrative of a larger community of persons who do not abandon us in our sufferings even though they cannot finally explain either our sufferings or their fidelity to us as we suffer.

Whether or not they have used the language of happiness and holiness, most Methodist theologians have remained within the boundaries suggested by the two themes: suffering is not a good but it need not be a meaningless absurdity. Such a theology of suffering has appeared in diverse forms, for example, among recent black Methodist theologians. James H. Cone, who began his religious reflections about suffering when he was a child in a small African Methodist Episcopal church in Arkansas, has argued that white theologians have been unduly preoccupied with the philosophical problem of evil—the problem of rationally reconciling the existence of an omnipotent and benevolent God with the continued reality of evil—and insufficiently attentive to the everyday suffering of oppressed people. The biblical account of suffering, he wrote, was not a philosophical account of the origin of evil but a proclamation about a God whose identity with the suffering of the world was revealed on a cross: "The cross of Jesus reveals the extent of God's involvement in the suffering of the weak."[39]

Cone insisted, though, that the crucifixion and resurrection of Jesus had nothing to do with resignation and the passive acceptance of suffering; the cross promised instead the liberation of the oppressed "from social and political bondage." For Cone, therefore, suffering as a medical issue could never be separated from suffering as a political and social reality, and he would contend that the Church seriously addresses the problem of suffering only when it struggles for a just social order in which proper medical care would be considered the right of every person. For Cone, a theology that remained faithful to the pain and hope of that African Methodist Episcopal congregation in a small Arkansas town could speak truly about medicine and health only insofar as it attended to the medical needs of poor black children and the physical pain of bodies broken by the misery of the ghetto. To assert that suffering is a good, Cone has written, is to run the risk of justifying the suffering borne by blacks. But to assert that suffering is utterly meaningless is to forsake the faith that had enabled blacks to endure, and to abandon the effort to overcome the sufferings that could be overcome.[40]

A related point of view can be seen in the *Manifesto a la Nación* which the Methodist Church of Bolivia published in 1970.

> Social, political, cultural, or economic structures become dehumanized when they do not serve "all men and the total man," in other words, when they are structured to perpetuate injustice. Structures are products of men, but they assume an impersonal character, even a Satanic one, going beyond the possibility of individual action.

Among an impoverished people, depressed by incredible unemployment, the Bolivians declared, a serious commitment to relieve suffering, including the physical suffering of the sick, will require that one attend to political tasks.[41]

Few Methodist theologians today attempt to explain and justify the reality of suffering. Many would hesitate to write a rational theodicy that presumed to offer an explanation for the suffering with which doctors and nurses, chaplains and pastors, patients and families struggle each day. They would prefer, rather, to return to the image of the suffering God. That image has appeared in a wide range of Methodist theologies. Edwin Lewis of Drew University wrote in the 1930s about the suffering of God in the tragedy of the cross. Georgia Harkness of Garrett Biblical Institute wrote in the 1940s about the meaning of the cross as the central Christian symbol: "whatever happens to [us]," she said, "God suffers most." William Strawson of Handsworth College wrote in the 1960s that Christians did not think of God as sending evil and suffering upon men and women as a punishment, but as assuming human nature and undergoing the "pains and sufferings of human life."[42]

Most Wesleyan theologians, therefore, would return, albeit with a different vocabulary, to Wesley's themes of happiness and holiness.

## SOME MEDICAL IMPLICATIONS

The conjunction of the two themes bears a certain pertinence for the dilemmas that occur daily in medical centers, dilemmas about abortion, about the delivery of an infant with severe birth defects, or about a suffering patient's desire for the cessation of pain through euthanasia. The Methodist tradition does not "solve" such dilemmas. It often speaks about them with a hesitant and divided voice. But it does assert that the avoidance of suffering is not the sole consideration in making judgments about them. The absence of suffering is a good, but it is not the only good, and it is not always the richest good. Far worse than the presence of suffering is the absence of love.

Wesley's two themes suggest that we are not to avoid suffering at all costs. They remind us, in fact, that we often cannot avoid suffering at all. Medical practice, even in its most sophisticated forms, will create suffering even as it tries to relieve it. The theologian Stanley Hauerwas has drawn from this fact an apt conclusion: we are not to manipulate our language to avoid recognizing the tragic character of medicine. We are not to say that "it is a good thing that we let the child die." It is far better, because more truthful, for us to say, if we must let the child die, that we faced a dilemma in which no "good" was available to us. We acted as we thought best; our act was nevertheless wrong; and we repent, even though we know that we will so act again, because we will face other decisions in which the good cannot be attained. But we will not deceive ourselves by speaking of a "good," for self-deception is the beginning of a moral insensitivity that can fail to recognize the good even when it can be attained.[43]

The boundaries established by the two Wesleyan themes also set certain salutary limits to our questions about terminating suffering by turning off the machines that keep us alive (or that prolong our suffering when it is merely a part of our dying). In saying that the Wesleyan insights set limits, I do not suggest that they solve the dilemma, but they do rule out two hasty and facile solutions. They preclude the ethical possibility of prolonging the suffering on the grounds that the suffering itself is somehow beneficial or that the suffering is not to be taken into account in making the decision. They preclude also the possibility of foreshortening the suffering on the grounds that the cessation of suffering is the only value to be considered. Between those two limits, a variety of other considerations might lead to a decision either to turn off the machine or to keep it on. But the two boundaries serve as reminder of the complexity and inevitable ambiguity that must be faced if the decision is to be morally responsible.

Hauerwas has also taken up an issue analogous to Wesley's concern about madness and mental and emotional suffering. In the decision to give birth to a child whom they know to be retarded, a family encounters directly a decision about unavoidable suffering. A decision to abort the birth brings suffering; a decision to have the child brings suffering. For Hauerwas, the dilemma raises larger questions about why we have children, in any case, and he usefully uncovers the hidden motive that often lies behind our decision to begin a family: the desire to reproduce ourselves and reach our unattained goals through our children. Driven by such a desire, we require that they be perfect in body and mind and that they realize our ideals and thereby justify our decision. In short, we often appeal in a shortsighted manner to only one side of the Wesleyan polarity: we are not here to suffer. And the matter therefore seems quite simple.

If we are to have children, though, because we are pledged to exist as a Christian community, Hauerwas wrote, and if we recognize that any child is a gift, not a construction of our ingenuity, then we might see and love the retarded child as a graphic embodiment of the truth that children are gifts who are not at our disposal. And if the avoidance of suffering is not the only good, we cannot automatically, as a matter of course, choose the easier way. It is always possible that a parent's love for a retarded child, within a community that draws the child into its life and maintains a place for the child in its communal story, signifies a possibility beyond that of dealing with suffering solely by eliminating it without regard for any other values. In short, the other side of the Wesleyan polarity—the assertion that suffering need not be utterly meaningless—balances and checks the prior assertion that we are not here to suffer. Again, the recognition of the boundaries by no means provides easy solutions. But it does reflect a communal narrative and a set of communal assumptions that help us deal honestly with the questions rather than prematurely choose either suffering or happiness for its own sake, as if love were without its own complicated inner dialectic of happiness and holiness.[44]

The Wesleyan dialectic not only serves the purpose of setting boundaries for ethical reflection, but it also helps to maintain a measure of realism in our attempts to define and understand the meaning of health. To say that we are not here to suffer is to imply an understanding of health as the absence of suffering. But to observe that suffering need not be utterly meaningless is to recognize that some forms of suffering and some forms of health can in fact coexist. The Methodist ethicist J. Robert Nelson has written of the diverse forms of suffering:

> There is suffering that seems cruel, destructive of life, and unbearable. There is suffering that seems grave only because we lack the courage or stamina to bear it. There is suffering accepted and endured out of respect or love for another person, for an idea, a cause or a faith. So there are varieties of suffering: some are clearly evil, some are beneficial, some are morally ambiguous. The wisdom of Christian faith counsels neither resignation to suffering nor avoidance of it. It teaches patience and endurance where suffering is inevitable, and willingness to suffer when it is altruistic and vicarious. The prime symbol of faith is the cross, representing divine suffering in the person of Jesus Christ on behalf of humanity.[45]

As a contrast to that recognition of suffering, Nelson noted the widespread Western ideal of health as a state of complete physical, mental, and social well-being, or the even more expansive ideal of health, proposed by a medical committee of the World Council of Churches, as "a dynamic state of well-being of the individual and of the society; of physical, mental, spiritual, economic, political and social well-being; of being in harmony with each other, with the material environment, and with God."[46]

One of the risks of such an expansive definition of health, as Nelson observes, is that "if health means everything good in life it really means nothing in particular."[47] An equally questionable implication is that every form of suffering, even the suffering undertaken on behalf of others, would seem to become a form of illness. In a hedonistic culture, the temptation is to assume that the voluntary acceptance of suffering, whether in moral commitment or in spiritual discipline, must cloak a hidden pattern of psychiatric distress, which would go away under the skillful ministrations of the therapist. And of course it might. But medicine cannot resolve every form of suffering, and not every instance of suffering can be reduced to a medical issue.

In the Christian journey, as the Wesleyan tradition has described it, suffering is a barrier. We are not here to suffer. But insofar as suffering enhances the capacity to love, it bears a meaning. Methodists have often been tempted to overstate its meaning, to call for resignation as an ethical duty. Our current temptation, it seems, is to deny altogether its meaning, to call for medication as a quick solution to every form of suffering, even the suffering that earlier generations might have understood as profound spiritual anguish. The Wesleyan tradition offers no simple solution to the problem of suffering, whether of the body or of the spirit. Clearly it calls for opposition to every form of needless and involuntary suffering; clearly it calls for a sympathetic and unflinching recognition of the power and reality of suffering; clearly it urges us to remain aware that even within the communities of healing suffering will remain as a tragic signature of our finitude. And it provides some useful boundaries for ethical and religious reflection. But it also recognizes that much of our suffering remains unclear, that we see it as in a mirror darkly, and that we often make our way through the darkness of the journey in hope and love more than in wisdom and knowledge.

# ·4·

# Dying and Death

Wesley always believed that the Christian should have no fear of death. To cower from death or to grieve for the dead was, he thought, to exemplify the sinfulness to which human nature was captive. The Christian would accept death with trust and resignation: "He cannot fear death; being able to trust Him he loves with his soul as well as his body; yea, glad to leave the corruptible body in the dust, till it is raised incorruptible and immortal." When the time came for Wesley to die, he maintained the faith. On his deathbed, he awoke and softly sang a stanza of one of his favorite hymns: "I'll praise my Maker while I've breath, and when my voice is lost in death, Praise shall employ my nobler power." The next day Wesley underwent the death for which he had hoped.[1]

Yet he did not always maintain his calm in the face of death. He once confided to his journal that although he approved of resignation and submission in death, he found in himself no capacity for either. He feared death. He often returned to the theme: "Let death look me in the face, and my spirit is troubled. Nor can I say, 'To die is gain.'" During his voyage to Georgia in 1735, Wesley was awed by the courage of a Moravian band aboard the ship during a frightening storm, for he recognized himself to be terrified at the thought of death at sea. More than three decades later, he revealed in a letter to his brother Charles a continuing sense of anxiety: "If I have any fear," he wrote, "it is not that of falling into hell but of falling into nothing." The fear of death was the mark of a fallen creation, and Wesley recognized that he, and everyone else, shared in the burdens of that fallen creation, including the burden of fearfulness in the face of death.[2]

His conflicting attitudes toward dying and death reflected his theological convictions. His theology could account for both the grieving and the singing, the trust and the fear. As the Methodist tradition changed, the theologians tried to maintain that balance. But the passions of living and dying often have a way of spilling over theological boundaries, and Methodists have exhibited a broad range of attitudes toward death and dying.

Christians who now live and worship within the Methodist tradition—whether they view themselves, in our hackneyed categories, as "liberal" or "conservative"—sometimes find it difficult to retain Wesley's certainties. Consider, for example, his sermon for the funeral of a youth named John Griffith, preached when Wesley was a young man. He used the occasion to comment on the sinfulness of profuse sorrowing for the dead. "Why should I be so unreasonable, so unkind, as to desire the return of a soul now in happiness to me?" he asked the grieving family. All occasions, he told them, must be borne with patience and moderation. Grief that impaired the rational faculties was "absurd, unprofitable, and sinful."[3]

It is worth remembering that Wesley preached the sermon in 1726, when he was still confiding in his journal his own secret fears of death, and that such sermons were common in the eighteenth century. We see him as something other than merely an insensitive young prig when we see the sermon as either an eighteenth-century convention or an expression of his inner anguish. Even the most traditional Methodist today would probably agree that a funeral sermon seems an inappropriate occasion to inform a family that immoderate grief would reveal their absurdity and sinfulness.

Taken as a whole, however, Wesley's theology formulated a useful set of images that have endured throughout the history of the tradition and offered helpful boundaries for continued reflection on the topics of dying and death. Wesley envisioned all of life as surrounded by the horizon of death. That recognition itself can be of service in an era that either hides the reality of death, disguising it within romantic wishfulness, or views it as unmitigated evil.[4]

Methodist theology has also returned repeatedly to another set of images that Wesley used to interpret dying and death: the images of penalty and promise. To view the themes of penalty and promise as standing in tension with each other within the larger theme of journeying offers a useful insight into the way the Methodist tradition has for almost three centuries understood the mysteries of death.

## PENALTY AND PROMISE

Wesley maintained throughout his adult life a consistent vision of death as both penalty and promise. The tension between the two descriptions enabled him to avoid either the sentimental illusion that death was painless and unreal or the despairing illusion that no hope and possibility could stand before the power of death. The Methodist tradition has tended to favor the view of death as promise. In recent decades, however, Methodist theologians and ethicists have begun to recover the other view: the theme of death as penalty, in whatever form or vocabulary it might find expression, seems necessary as an ethical reminder that our attempts to control and manipulate death are properly limited.

When Wesley conceived of death as a penalty, he was thinking of a Christian tradition that interpreted death as punishment for the sin in the garden. According to Wesley's reading of the Scripture, the fall into sinfulness brought temporal, spiritual, and eternal death, and all three dimensions of death were to be viewed as punishment. As a result, Wesley viewed death as an enemy, a punitive and relentless adversary that visited each generation, and he insisted that such a view of death be retained within Christian piety.

In 1738, the Unitarian John Taylor of Norwich scandalized the orthodox, including Wesley, by writing a treatise denying the doctrine of original sin. He insisted as part of his argument that although temporal death might be considered a consequence of the Fall, death "spiritual and eternal" should not be. Taylor's point was that spiritual and eternal death resulted from sinful choices, not from a sinful condition rooted in an original sin.

Wesley believed that the universality of divine grace solved the problem of original sin, but he felt that Taylor's treatise, by calling into question the doctrine of original sin, threatened to subvert the Christian understanding of redemption. He also thought that Taylor had grievously misunderstood the problem of death. The ensuing debate between the two men clarified two important issues in Wesley's understanding of death.

First, Taylor would acknowledge that temporal death was a consequence of the sin in the garden, but he would not speak of it as a "punishment" for that sin. One reason for his reluctance was that Taylor viewed temporal death as a "benefit" for humanity. He thought that it encouraged men and women to think about serious matters, and it served for Christians as the entrance to heaven. In Taylor's theology, death became, in more ways than one, an elevating and ennobling experience, a benefit to the soul.

Wesley disagreed. "Death is not properly a benefit," he said, "but a punishment." In the best of all possible worlds, he thought, death perhaps ought to be viewed as a benefit, but he doubted the actual benefits of death in eighteenth-century England. On the whole, he wrote, the thought of death did not elevate the soul to nobler truths. On the whole, the more men and women thought about death, the more terrifying and burdensome they found it, and the more they clung to the pleasures of the transitory world. To reduce the matter to its simplest terms, Wesley thought it somewhat silly to conceive of death as "good" rather than "bad."[5]

Second, Taylor wanted to define temporal death as simply as possible. Thus he took a step in the direction of defining death merely as the cessation of biological function. To Wesley it seemed that the simplifying was excessive. For him, death was infinitely more complicated; it was a complex reality permeated with the residues of all human history and signaling an end to all merely human possibility. Its implications stretched from the garden to the final judgment. Temporal death was so closely interwoven with spiritual death and eternal death that it defied every effort to reduce it merely to biological terms. Even as a temporal event, death broke through all narrow definitions. Death for Wesley was a terrifying and awesome reality that implied "all manner of evils, to which either the body or the soul is liable."[6]

Wesley saw no incongruity, therefore, in the Christian's acknowledging the inevitability of death and yet struggling against it. He offered his approval and support for the English "Humane Society" that formed to study the means of restoring to life persons apparently struck with sudden death. The society continued the work of similar groups that had begun in 1700 in Holland to try to resuscitate apparent victims of drowning or other accidents. To Wesley, its work exemplified the power that God had entrusted to humanity. "See with what wisdom he had endued these sons of mercy! Teaching them to stop the parting soul, to arrest the spirit just quitting the breathless clay, and taking wing for eternity." Because he refused to view death as a benefit, Wesley could consistently support the battle against death.[7]

Because he saw death as inevitable, Wesley urged physicians to recognize and accept their limits. He thought it beyond the capacity of the doctor to overcome the power of death. "Be men ever so great masters of the art of healing, can they prevent or heal the gradual decays of nature? Can all their boasted skill heal old age or hinder dust from returning to dust? Nay, who, among the greatest masters of medicine, has been able to add a century to his own years?"[8] His reservation could be interpreted as a taunt against medical pretension. It could also be interpreted as a gentle reminder that physicians need not assume the responsibility for burdens that lie beyond their reach. As a divine punishment, death resisted our best effort to overcome it. But to the doctor tempted to assume the burden of God, Wesley thought, the divine No could also be read as a divine Yes of forgiveness and freedom from an unrealistic expectation.

By viewing death as penalty and punishment, Wesley avoided the sentimental assessment of dying as merely the completion and fulfillment of human growth, or as simply a natural event, to be accepted and celebrated as the completion of a natural process. No doubt, to later generations of Methodists, the language of punishment and penalty has seemed more a characteristic of scholastic debate than a useful means of interpreting dying and death. Few Methodist theologians now speak of penalty and punishment when they speak of death. Nevertheless, Methodists have not entirely forgotten one of Wesley's main points: Death is not a benefit and not simply a biological fact. Its meaning is far richer, and far more terrible, than that.

Wesley also believed that death contained a promise. He believed in both the immortality of the soul and the resurrection of the body. The soul, he said, did not die; hence the "moment the breath of man goeth forth, he is an inhabitant of eternity." In death, the souls of the faithful transcended the limits imposed by the body and entered into an "intermediate state" of increasing sanctification and praise. Their bodies returned to the dust, to await recomposition and transformation on the great Day of the Lord when Jesus would return to judge the quick and the dead. On that day, the glorified bodies of the faithful would rise in power, glory, and spirit, and dwell, reunited with their souls, in an invisible world. On that same day, the souls and bodies of the faithless would reunite in an endless and fiery hell.[9]

Because death contained the promise of life in another world, Wesley assumed that the ideal death would be "a calm passage out of life, full of even, rational peace and joy." For the Christian "to die was gain," so he felt disappointed when Methodists were "uneasy at the apprehension of death." He filled his journals with deathbed accounts, and he clearly admired any sign of resignation and acceptance among dying Christians. He wanted them to "give thanks in everything" and to "praise God with every breath." A woman named Betty Fairbridge, for example, enjoyed, in Wesley's view, an ideal death: "But her bodily weakness increased: so much the more did her faith and love increase; till prayer was swallowed up in praise, and she went away with triumphant joy." John Bennets also had a good death: "A little before his death, he examined each of his children concerning their abiding in the faith. Being satisfied of this, he told them, 'Now I have no doubt but that we shall meet again at the right hand of our Lord.' He then cheerfully committed his soul to him, and fell asleep." But a "rich man in London" suffered a bad death. "When the physician told him, 'He must die,' [he] gnashed his teeth, and clenched his fist, and cried out vehemently, 'God, God, I won't die!' But he died with the very words in his mouth. And was buried; doubtless with pomp enough, suitably to his quality."[10]

For Wesley, the promise of death was the promise of a future life of happiness and praise. He believed in the promise so intensely that in reading his sermons and his accounts of death among the pious, one almost loses sight of the duality in his view of dying and death. The sober assessment of death as penalty, as punishment, as a frightening prospect, fades into the background of the death narratives, and with its fading the complicated richness of Wesley's imagery also flattens into an optimism that fails to convey the complexity even of his own thought and experience.

For this and other reasons, the history of the Methodist tradition throughout the first century and a half after Wesley's death in 1791 was a story of ever-increasing insistence on the promise. Only with the appearance of new and remarkable life-saving techniques and technologies after the Second World War did Methodist theologians emphasize once again that the maintaining of a humane society, and of a Christian ministry to the dying, might well require a balanced view of death as both promise and penalty.

## DEATH AS PROMISE

Throughout the early nineteenth century, Methodists retained the dual sense of death as both penalty and promise. Richard Watson wrote that death was the "penalty of disobedience," and he claimed that the Scripture presented it as temporal, spiritual, and eternal. But he also thought that sanctified Christians enjoyed a victory over death that freed them from fear and permitted them a spirit of calm acceptance: "A patient resignation to the will of God, as to the measure of their bodily sufferings, and the strong hopes and joyful anticipations of a better life, cancel and subdue that horror of pain and dissolution which is natural to man."[11]

Watson's own death became exemplary for nineteenth-century Methodists, precisely because it illustrated the struggle for resignation that would be expected of a Christian who recognized death as both penalty and promise. During the early stages of his death, he had frequent recourse to a familiar saying from an earlier Anglican worthy: "Since I owe thee a death, Lord, let it not be terrible, and then take thine own time; I submit to it. Let not mine, O Lord, but let thy will be done." He did not simply assume that he would be properly submissive. He recognized "how much labor and pain it costs to unroof this house; to take down this tabernacle and tent," and he feared that he would succumb to "agony and struggle in his last moments." At the same time, Watson urged his family to compose themselves, keep their minds calm, and commit the matter to God. He discussed his death with visitors and made careful arrangements for it; he offered numerous testimonies to divine mercy; and he died with calm and composure.[12]

The dual depiction of death deeply informed Methodist devotional writings throughout the early nineteenth century. Methodists could speak of death as "appalling," as the "king of terrors," evoking in every man and woman the "solemn consciousness of a common doom." They recognized the "effort of mankind to repress the consciousness of the fact," as if forgetfulness could "forestall its inexorable approach." They did not hesitate to speak of death as an "awful reality." Nevertheless, they urged Christians to remain always mindful of death, never allowing themselves to be "carried along in the current of life, heedless of all things except the transient passing stream." The "genuine Christian," wrote the American Methodist Abel Stevens, contemplated death "more or less habitually." The Christian, he said, "lives for death." And the ground of that capacity to live for death was the promise of life with Christ. Fortified with the promise, the Christian could achieve the final "victory" over death, could defeat the enemy.[13]

Wesleyan theologians produced a considerable number of devotional treatises on dying and death. In early Methodist memoirs and journals, a third or more of the total narrative might be occupied by an account of the final week of life, and the ideal was submissive resignation. A typical example can be found in the popular account of *The Experience and Gospel Labours of the Rev. Benjamin Abbott*, who was an ordinary traveling preacher in Pennsylvania and New York in the late eighteenth century. His biographer described his death for the edification of other Methodists:

> During the day he continued in a rack of excruciating pain, which he bore with a christian patience and resignation. He was happy in God, and rejoiced at his approaching dissolution, and seemed much engaged in his soul with God. He appeared to possess his rational faculties to his last moments; and for some time previous thereunto he was delivered from excruciating pain, to the joy of his friends; his countenance continued joyful, heavenly, and serene. His last sentence that was intelligibly articulated was, Glory to God! I see heaven sweetly opening before me! After this, his speech so much failed, that he could not be distinctly understood, only now and then a word, as, see! see! glory! glory! . . . The sting of death was plucked out; and death came as a messenger of peace to him.[14]

In such early Methodist writings, the accent fell on the duty of resignation and acceptance. But the writers recognized that resignation was no easy achievement. Despite the moralism with which they urged resignation, they understood that death was no simple promise. It was also punishment and penalty, and hence an awesome task.[15]

Toward the end of the nineteenth century, Methodists began to minimize the terrors of death. The theologians, to be sure, continued to write of death as both penalty and promise. The theologian William Burt Pope, for example, a native of Nova Scotia who became a tutor at Didsbury College in England and the most important English Methodist theologian of the later nineteenth century, published in 1875 a three-volume *Compendium of Christian Theology* that explicated the standard Methodist doctrine. In it he explained death—"a word of large meaning in theology"—as both "the penalty of human sin" and a "departure from this life to another." He considered death a probationary discipline, indeed, the last event in the probation of the fallen creature, as well as a form of Christian obedience and martyrdom, hallowed and dignified as part of the Christian's fellowship with the dying Christ.[16]

In popular Wesleyan piety, however, a new attitude toward death had by 1875 already begun to appear. Wesleyan journalists began to deplore the excesses of the older deathbed piety, which they viewed as unduly productive of "terror," and to place their accent on "hope." They discouraged intrusive curiosity about the last words of the dying. "We are to be judged by how we have lived," wrote one Methodist, "and not by how we have died." And they assured the dying that it was all right for them simply to die quietly, without feeling any guilt about their inability to "enter with intense earnestness into the prayers offered in the sick room."[17]

In place of the older devotional writings on dying and death, they produced new devotional articles on the joys of immortality. They described heavenly existence in copious detail and assured the dying that they would not only recognize their loved ones there but also share a continuing interest in everything that happened on earth.

> It is a cheering thought that when we die we shall be interested in all that is transpiring on this globe; that we shall know, far more intimately than we can now know, every event which is taking place here. Our vision is now limited. Then we shall embrace in one view all the nations, tribes, and families, from the equator to the pole.[18]

A piety of promise and cheer overwhelmed the earlier piety of resignation.[19]

The change can be traced in English Methodist hymnals. The 1874 edition of the hymnal added 30 new hymns on the future life, and by 1904, the Methodists in England decided to reduce dramatically the number of hymns on death and judgment. Whereas the 1874 hymnal contained 25 hymns about death, the 1904 hymnal contained 9. English Methodists in 1874 could sing as many as 19 hymns about the final judgment; in 1904 they could sing only 7. By 1933, the Methodists in England decided to reduce again the number of selections not only about death and judgment but also about the future life: the 1904 book contained 37 such hymns; the 1933 hymnal had only 19.[20]

The change appeared, as well, in the tone and the liturgy of Methodist funerals. In the eighteenth century funerals served as occasions for evangelistic sermons on the piety of the deceased and the terrors of death for the unconverted, and for singing processions designed as a witness to the community's faith. The congregation normally dressed in black attire, and the churches and chapels were sometimes draped in black cloth. (At Wesley's funeral, the executors chose a sturdy black cloth that could be given afterward to sixty poor women for clothing.) By the late nineteenth century, Methodist funerals began to assume a new tone. In 1884, Methodists in America added to the older funeral liturgy a prayer confirming the "joy and felicity" of the future life and asking for "perfect consummation and bliss, both in body and soul." By 1916, they deleted from the service older citations from the book of Job that had included the reminder that "worms destroy this body." They also declined to retain the older lament that "man that is born of woman hath but a short time to live, and is full of misery," and they omitted the older liturgical reference to the pains of death. Their "Order for the Burial of the Dead" contained a new selection of scriptural passages designed for consolation and comfort. Like other American Protestants, they also began to cast aside the black cloth of mourning and to conduct their funeral services in the midst of colorful flowers that symbolized faith and hope.[21]

By the late nineteenth century, moreover, Methodist theologians had become bold in their willingness to advance rational arguments for the doctrine of immortality. Richard Watson, in 1823, had devoted his attention to the "resurrection of the body," which he understood as a mystery hidden from reason and revealed only in Scripture. By 1847, the American Wesleyan theologian Thomas Ralston was contending that both reason and Scripture confirmed a Christian faith in the immortality of the soul. Through careful attention to the nature of human consciousness and the vast powers of the soul, he thought, the devout philosopher could produce rational evidence for the doctrine of immortality, even apart from the scriptural revelation.[22]

By 1894 John Miley, theologian at Drew Theological Seminary, was acknowledging that there were "few texts of Scripture in which our immortality is directly asserted," but also insisting that rational argument could demonstrate the doctrine and that its truth was presupposed throughout the Old and New Testaments. It was not surprising that Miley also denied the penal character of death and that he described the beauties of heaven in detail. By the late nineteenth century, a considerable number of Methodists would speak only of the promise implicit in death, not of its terrors.[23]

Throughout the early twentieth century, the standard Methodist doctrine was not resurrection but immortality, and theologians seemed convinced that rational arguments could at least exhibit the plausibility of the doctrine. The Boston personalist Albert C. Knudson, for example, viewed death as simply the "natural lot" of humanity rather than a penal event: "When it comes at the end of a long life," he wrote, "there is no complaint." Though he recognized the flaws in the standard arguments for immortality, Knudson insisted that the doctrine was an inevitable corollary of the Christian understanding of God as a holy, loving, omnipotent creator and redeemer. Georgia Harkness at Garrett Biblical Institute concurred: "Were there no other reason for believing in immortality," she wrote, "the goodness of God is reason enough."[24]

It is not surprising, then, that a firm confidence in life after death has been a hallmark of Wesleyan piety in the twentieth century. In 1962, at least 86 percent of the Methodists in the United States insisted that a belief in life after death was essential for Christians who would maintain a strong sense of social responsibility, and undoubtedly a larger percentage accepted the doctrine of immortality without holding any opinion about its relationship to social responsibility. Only about 3 percent indicated any skepticism about the doctrine. At the same time, twentieth-century Methodists had departed from the tendency of their nineteenth-century forebears to think of salvation as a matter of "going to heaven and escaping hell." Only about 2 percent of American Methodists entertained such a notion of salvation. More than 90 percent thought of salvation as either peace and joy with God through forgiveness or the power to live a new life in fellowship with God and neighbor. In that respect, twentieth-century American Methodists retained an identifiably Wesleyan conception of salvation, while they had moved quite a distance from the traditional Wesleyan understanding of death as both penalty and promise. The sense of death as promise had overwhelmed the notion of death as penalty.[25]

The Wesleyan tradition has, however, in recent years recovered something of the inner meaning of the older duality in the theological interpretation of death. The appropriation of the older sensibility has gone largely unobserved, because the traditional language, especially the language of "penalty" and "punishment," has fallen into disuse. Nevertheless, the theologians who worked most closely with issues of dying and death found that a simple accent on the promise masked the realities that they were encountering. They came to recognize that an adequate understanding of death requires a sympathetic awareness that most Christians do not view death as a friend but as an enemy.

## PENALTY AND PROMISE REVISITED

The recovery and reinterpretation of the older sensibility became visible primarily among pastoral theologians and ethicists. The pastoral theologians recognized the need to be present with the dying and to take into account their own perceptions of what was happening to them. They therefore discovered anew that the dying rarely viewed their death simply as promise; they felt it as penalty, as an alien imposition. The ethicists recognized the dilemmas—and the temptations—of the physicians and families who cared for the dying. They therefore discovered anew the dangers of viewing death simply as promise; they saw the need to emphasize also its character as penalty.

Such abstractions assume concrete shape for the theologian through the biblical story of creation and fall in Genesis. In the biblical account, death came of disobedience: "You may freely eat of every tree of the garden, but of the tree of the knowledge of good and evil you shall not eat, for in the day that you eat of it you shall die"(Genesis 2:16). So spoke the Lord God to the Man. But the Man and the Woman ate of the forbidden fruit when they accepted the promise of the serpent: "You will not die. . . . You will be like God, knowing good and evil" (Genesis 3:4–5). The result was the curse of the Lord God: "You are dust, and to dust you shall return" (Genesis 3:19). But God did not then abandon the Man and the Woman. God remained with them and entered into covenant with their heirs and promised to be their God even as they returned to the dust.

When Paul wrote his letter to the Romans, he returned to this story to interpret for them the death of Christ: As sin and death came into the world through the transgression in the garden, so forgiveness and life came through the obedience on the cross. Through the life and death of Jesus Christ, the promise overcame the penalty (Romans 5:6–21). Yet Paul knew that he lived not simply within the realm of life and the promise but also within the realm of death and the penalty: "Wretched man that I am!" he wrote. "Who will deliver me from the body of death?" (Romans 8:24).

In attempting to interpret the story of creation, fall, and redemption, Methodist theologians retained the themes of penalty and promise. They did so not simply as a gesture to tradition; they saw that both dimensions of the story seemed to interpret their own living and dying.

For them, to speak of death as penalty was to assert that death was not to be simply accepted as the natural aim of creation. God breathed the breath of life, not of death, into the Man and the Woman. God commanded them to avoid the tree that brought death. They returned to the dust only because they disobeyed the command. Traditional Methodist theologians always assumed that they would have lived forever had they not disobeyed. Hence the tradition has been uneasy with the claim that death is merely a natural event, to be accepted as part of God's intention. To seek God's intention, the Methodist tradition looked to the garden—and death did not dwell in the garden. Hence death is not to be accepted; death is to be fought.

In the Methodist tradition, however, death is not interpreted as a final victory of the serpent. For Methodist theologians, to speak of death as promise was to assert that death was not to be simply resisted as if it represented only the domain of evil. God entered into a covenant of life, not of death, with the heirs of the Man and the Woman, inviting them to trust in the cross that brought life. Traditional Methodist theologians claimed that the trustful would live in God. Hence the tradition has been uneasy with the claim that death is sheer evil, to be resisted as the utter collapse of God's intention. To seek God's intention, the Methodist tradition looked to the cross—and the cross transformed the meaning of death. Hence death is not to be resisted at any cost; death is not to be fought indefinitely.

To speak of death as a penalty, moreover, is to acknowledge that we do not view death as a "solution" properly subject to our control. It is a problem, not a solution; a mystery, not an answer. Because we encounter death as penalty, it eludes our control. It is not ours to use as a means. It is not ours, ultimately, to understand or to manage or to overcome. To speak of death as promise, though, is also to affirm that we do not view death as so alien and so problematic and so elusive that we must remain still and dumb in its presence.

Whenever they have spoken in language that suggests penalty and promise, Methodist theologians have echoed a larger biblical story and affirmed it as their story. Their care for the dying has been informed by their sense of location within that larger narrative. But one must be careful not to assume that living from within the biblical story is the same as having clear rules to govern every decision. If we look to the Methodist tradition for precise guidance on medical procedures with the dying, we look in vain. A religious tradition is not a substitute for painstaking ethical reflection. Yet the painstaking reflection, however abstract and secular it might appear, almost always bears a trace of a larger religious vision, however dim it might be. And in drawing the outlines of the larger vision, the historian can often clarify the boundaries within which ethical and pastoral decisions are made.

The renewed sensitivity to the dual dimension of death appeared first among the Methodist pastoral theologians. In 1936, the Methodist chaplain Russell Dicks urged pastors who ministered to the sick and dying to start where people "really were." He recorded one of his own pastoral conversations with a patient who was believed to be dying: "She said, 'I think I am going to die.' I said, 'You are not afraid, are you?' After considering, she said, 'No, I am not afraid.'" And that, said Dicks, "is starting with a patient where you find her, and moving at once toward the point which the patient needs to reach."[26]

Dicks's response was, in fact, an appeal to the woman's will, an appeal to the will to reach an exceedingly difficult goal. And such an appeal underlay all of Dicks's reflections on dying. In 1941 he was claiming that religion was concerned not with how long a person lived but with how a person died. When he published in 1953 a popular devotional guide on dying and death, he advocated a "heroic" death that seemed reminiscent of a nineteenth-century ideal: "I further believe that the human creature is capable of a heroic death. While most people die commonplace deaths, with vision clouded and hope dimmed, little realizing and seemingly not caring what is happening to them, this need not be."[27] Dicks proposed a series of devotional "exercises" in which the living could imagine their dying, assuming, one supposes, that devotional techniques could overcome the alien power. In that respect, Dicks retained the attitudes of the late nineteenth-century theologians who inaugurated flower-bedecked funerals and encouraged cheerfulness as a means of promoting heroic confidence among Christians.

Even so, as his conversation with the dying woman might also suggest, Dicks did urge pastors to look at the reality of death. He did not immediately reassure her—in order to reassure himself—that her anticipation of her death was surely mistaken, and he did not change the topic. In that moment of pastoral conversation, therefore, one can see the beginning, however shadowy, of the recovery of an older recognition that death can appear to the dying as punishment and penalty and that their perception of it as penalty may be closer to its religious meaning than would be a one-sided perception of it as promise.

When Paul Johnson of Boston University provided guidance in 1953 for pastors ministering to the dying, he cautioned them that death was no "ordinary event"; it bore within itself the "forces of destruction." Johnson hastened to add that the pastor brought to the dying "the historic affirmation of the Christian faith that God cares for every life and will lead this person across the threshold of death to a life beyond," but his attention to the terrifying mystery of death signaled a new willingness on the part of pastoral theologians to stand with the dying in their darkness. They prepared the way for the later insistence by Methodist pastoral theologians that pastors and physicians recognize the "anguish" of death.[28]

Charles Gerkin of Emory University represented that emerging sensibility when he spoke in 1979 of death as a "narrowing, strangling experience that has about it a certain angry torment." Gerkin warned against the temptation to offer reassurance instead of standing with the dying as they entered the tight, angry, and terrifying darkness. What the dying often fear most, he observed, was abandonment and forsakenness. Ministers or physicians who wished to embody the presence of the incarnate Christ would stand by the dying in their suffering, while also remaining aware that they stood outside that suffering and could therefore do nothing to prevent it, whether by offering words of reassurance or by holding out false hopes.[29]

It was to be expected that Methodists, whose tradition speaks of stages and levels of Christian holiness, would be attracted to the argument that even the dying normally come to terms with their death in recognizable stages or levels. Elisabeth Kübler-Ross won considerable attention from Methodists when she argued that the dying often proceeded through five stages: denial, anger, bargaining with death, depression, and final acceptance of the inevitability and appropriateness of death.[30]

Not all Methodist theologians liked the proposal. Some insisted that a prescriptive application of the theory can provide simply one more means of abandoning the dying by imposing deceptive expectations on them. To use traditional Wesleyan language: because death is penalty as well as promise, it eludes our efforts at control and management, as well as our presumption that we can understand and explain. To speak of stages of dying may well become one more instance, however well-meaning, of our presumption that the promise is ours to bestow. "If I wish to die without reaching the stage of 'acceptance,'" wrote Stanley Hauerwas, "that is my right, whether others think I am dying a 'good death' or not." "I prefer," he added, "the realism of the New Testament."[31]

The reappropriation of a sense of death as penalty has not signaled any abandonment of the affirmation that death is also promise. For one thing, the theologians recognize that death can come as a welcome friend after a long life or an extended period of intolerable suffering. For another, they know that it can be grasped as an occasion for participation, not only in the death of Christ on the cross but also in the community of love that surrounds the dying. For still another, they have insisted that it does not inevitably overcome the "trust of God's promise of the ultimate coming together of all things, that hope which has since Paul been called the hope of the resurrection."[32] The Methodist tradition, now as in the past, speaks pastorally of the promise, though now, as in the past, it speaks of the promise from within an awareness of death as penalty.

Sensitivity to this duality has been especially prominent among the Methodist ethicists who have reflected on the moral dilemmas that accompany care for the dying. To think of death as penalty is to recognize that death is to be fought; to think of it as promise is to recognize that it is not to be fought indefinitely. The danger of forgetting its character as penalty is that we abandon prematurely the struggle against death. The danger of forgetting its character as promise is that we shall compel the dying to prolong their dying unnecessarily. The difficult task is to maintain the inner tension between the two visions of death, compelling the one always to confront the other.

The tension between the two is visible throughout recent ethical reflection among Methodist theologians on the quandaries of dying and death. The reflection has produced no unanimity within the tradition. It is impossible to speak of an official Methodist "position" about such topics as suicide, euthanasia, death with dignity, the cessation of life-maintaining medical support systems, and the problem of whether to use "extraordinary" or "heroic" means of sustaining life and fending off death. But Methodists have pondered the questions, and in the distant background of their debates one can see the dim outline of a larger theological understanding of death as penalty and promise.

Earlier generations of Methodists had no difficulty in affirming the traditional Christian prohibition of suicide. One of Wesley's less attractive moments came when he suggested, in his treatise on suicide, that the bodies of men and women who had killed themselves should be hung from chains in public places. Against the eighteenth-century English jurists who contended that suicide should be considered a sure evidence of madness, Wesley could only assert the prohibition and suggest a gruesome punishment for the dead.[33]

Later Methodists retained the prohibition, but with a greater measure of moderation than Wesley had managed to show. The nineteenth-century theologian Henry Bidleman Bascom argued against suicide on two grounds. The first was utilitarian: life should be preserved for its usefulness, and suicide defrauded the wider society of its rightful expectation that all of its members would remain useful as long as they could. The second was theological: a human life—including our own life—was the workmanship of God, a gift of God, and hence not ours, by right, to destroy.[34]

The consideration of suicide as an ethical problem in medicine usually occurs in relation to terminal illness. When patients undergo intolerable suffering and feel immeasurable despair about the burdens that their suffering or disability imposes—and will continue to impose—on their families and friends, Bascom's reminders about our obligations to remain socially useful seem pitifully inadequate. (One must recall, in fairness, that Bascom was not writing about the special case of the terminally ill.) Indeed any recital of legalistic prohibitions fails to recognize the ambiguities that overshadow a decision made by a person who in despair (and in despairing love for family and friends) seeks "to wrest a fragment of dignity from a life which has become impossible."[35] To the despairing among the terminally ill, suicide can indeed seem to offer a promise, however bleak, of release.

It yet remains true, for someone formed by the Methodist tradition, that suicide cannot be considered a fitting and appropriate means of bringing either suffering or life to a conclusion. The vision of death as penalty reminds us that death is to be fought and that the struggle against it is not to be abandoned prematurely. And suicide is almost always a premature abandonment of the struggle.

One says "almost always" in the recognition that no inflexible prohibition can guide decision in every dilemma. But the prohibition, however inflexibly and unfeelingly it might sometimes have been expressed, did embody a theological wisdom. Bascom did represent the wisdom of the tradition when he observed that Christians consider human life as a gift and not as our own achievement which we are free to prolong or destroy at will. Furthermore, the prohibition did reflect the awareness that suicide, at least in the culture formed by the Jewish and Christian past, remains always an ambiguous rejection not only of suffering but also of love.

The Methodist theologian James Laney makes the point in a way strikingly consonant with the Wesleyan claim that the struggle against death as penalty is not to be abandoned prematurely. He suggests that suicide is almost always a premature abandonment of life precisely because the struggle against death is always undertaken within the bonds of community, especially of community with those whom we love and who love us. And insofar as our suicide—even the suicide performed with the intent of relieving their suffering—destroys a bond that helped to sustain their own common struggle against the powers of death, then suicide destroys something precious.

Suicide, he observes, almost always represents, however subtly, "a judgment not only upon the uselessness of the life taken, but upon the supporting fabric" provided by a larger community of family and friends.

> Even when explanatory notes are left behind, true motivation and intent remain shrouded in mystery, inviting interpretation. Suicide is inescapably unethical not only because it is a taking of life, but because it is invariably social. Suicide cannot but be a negative condemnation of the whole of life, and thus of the relations of those who live on after.[36]

Such an argument, one should note, assumes that friendship is itself a strong bond of mutual commitment and responsibility—an assumption hardly representative of fashionable expectations in Western culture about "mutually enhancing relationships." But it also suggests, in typical Methodist fashion, that death, as penalty, resists our efforts to control it, and that the effort to conquer it for the sake of beloved friends and family can also inadvertently destroy a precious hope and confidence that sustain the beloved as they remain by us in our (and in their) suffering.

Even more problematic is the issue of euthanasia, the painless inducement of death in patients suffering unbearable pain or existing in a comatose state within a terminal illness. The progress of medical technology has made the issue increasingly crucial and difficult, for our new machines, drugs, and surgical techniques can prolong biological life long beyond the time that patients wish to live. The dying, in fact, can reach the point of viewing the life-sustaining machines as exquisite instruments of torture, perversely binding them within their suffering. And the families of comatose patients can come to view them as troubling instruments, too, maintaining circulation and respiration within biological organisms long after the possibility of human access to loved ones has passed.

The Methodist tradition offers no binding rule that governs every painful decision. Yet Methodist theologians have been able to agree that involuntary euthanasia, the killing of patients who wish to live or express no desire to die, contradicts both the imperative of love and the Christian affirmation that life as a gift of God is sacred. For the same reason, they have been reluctant to approve the administration of death-inducing agents even to patients who request them. But they have been painfully aware of the danger that a refusal to grant the request might mean compelling the dying to prolong their dying unnecessarily.

A few Methodist theologians have questioned the traditional reluctance to grant such a request. The ethicist Harmon L. Smith of Duke University has suggested that the reluctance might cloak a refusal to accept moral responsibility for an ambiguous action that could yet be caring and ethically appropriate.

> Anyone familiar with the most rudimentary psychological insights will appreciate that a decision to terminate the life (and, incidentally, the pain) of an incurably diseased and distressed patient is equivocal and ambiguous. Similarly, anyone familiar with the most elementary ethical perceptions knows that no decision, and surely [no] one of great significance, is without doubt and risk. Families might be selfishly motivated; so may be doctors and nurses; even the patient himself may be pathologically depressed or crazed by pain. But a straightforward admission of these ingredients in the decision-making process does not prove 'beyond a reasonable doubt' that an intentional choice for death is a hateful and unloving act.[37]

Smith's suggestion is useful as a reminder that even refusal to grant the patient's request to receive death-inducing drugs can be ethically ambiguous. But Smith, like most other Methodist ethicists, is also reluctant to approve deliberate action calculated to cause death, even when death would come as a relief from suffering.[38]

The reluctance of Methodist ethicists to approve of direct euthanasia reflects, on one level, a wariness lest utilitarian criteria be accepted as normal warrants for medical practice. James Laney has written of the implicit danger in the question "Of what use is such a life?" Even to permit the question, he argues, is to enter "a realm of rational calculus which is fraught with peril." To justify the killing of the weak and the useless in any setting, but especially in such a setting as the hospital or clinic, is to repudiate the Christian regard for "the least of these." Paul Ramsey has cautioned against the acceptance of any practice that diminishes "medicine's impulse to save life," because for him that impulse embodies a covenant between physicians and patients, and a society which subverts that covenant also surrenders the trust that undergirds the practice of medicine.[39]

On another level, the reluctance to approve of direct euthanasia reflects an awareness of the moral ambiguity in the request of the dying patient or the patient's family. Have I the right to ask another person to assume the moral burden of killing me? Can I understand the burden of guilt that I might be imposing? Can I predict, within my suffering, how my loved ones will live with the memory of their involvement in my dying? Can I rightly ask the physician, committed to saving life, to assume the burden of taking mine? What responsibility do I have to other persons even as I suffer? Such questions serve again as a reminder that our death is social, and that its social meaning is most pronounced among those who care most for us. The theological assertion that death comes as penalty as well as promise entails the ethical claim that we are not to abandon prematurely the struggle against death. It is never easy to know what *premature* means in such a claim, but the recognition that our death is social suggests that we are usually abandoning the struggle prematurely if we must ask others to assume the burden of killing us.

Yet ethicists within the Wesleyan tradition, believing that death need not be fought indefinitely, have often maintained, implicitly or explicitly, the traditional Catholic moral distinction between killing a patient and permitting the dying patient to die, between commission and omission. Paul Ramsey has tried to chart a mediating path between the proponents of direct euthanasia and the advocates of medical scrupulosity who persist in efforts to save life regardless of the pain and agony they bring. "In omission," he argues, "no human agent causes the patient's death, directly or indirectly. He dies his own death from causes that it is no longer merciful or reasonable to fight by means of possible medical interventions." In arguing that it can be an act of mercy to withhold the treatment that artificially prolongs biological life, Ramsey expresses a position that is widely held among Methodists. The moment arrives when care for the dying means only caring for them as they are dying, rather than prolonging their dying.[40]

The proponents of euthanasia have argued that on the boundary lines of ethical decision the distinction between omission and commission evaporates. And Ramsey acknowledges such situations. When dealing with comatose patients who are, according to the best possible medical judgment, irretrievably inaccessible to human care, one might properly decide to inject an intravenous bubble of air. When dealing with a "prolonged dying in which it is medically impossible to keep severe pain at bay," one might properly decide to hasten the dying. Nonetheless, such exceptions to the general rule against the direct inducement of death, Ramsey argues, do not invalidate the rule.[41] And even Methodists who might disagree with Ramsey's conclusions have tended to find the distinction between omission and commission a useful guide, not because it establishes a fixed and static imperative, but because one purpose of such ethical distinctions is to enrich moral reflection by reminding us of complexities that we might otherwise forget.

The United Methodist Church in America has called in its statement of Social Principles for the acceptance in medical practice of "death with dignity."

> We applaud medical science for efforts to prevent disease and illness and for advances in treatment that extend the meaningful life of human beings. At the same time, in the varying stages of death and life that advances in medical science have occasioned, we recognize the agonizing personal and moral decisions faced by the dying, their physicians, their families, and their friends. Therefore, we assert the right of every person to die in dignity, with loving personal care and without efforts to prolong terminal illnesses merely because the technology is available to do so.[42]

The statement reflects the traditional Wesleyan assertion that death need not, indeed should not, be fought indefinitely. The theological understanding of death as promise leads to the ethical awareness that we abuse our medical knowledge when we use it to force upon another the "mere continuation of life in a biological sense."[43]

Yet the call for death with dignity threatens always to overstate the promise and gloss over the penal dimension of death. The rhetoric can suggest an image of a "good death" as rational, calm, controlled. Such deaths undoubtedly occur, and their occurrence is often cause for gratitude. But people who talk about death with dignity are also prone on occasion to speak of death as "beautiful," "glorious," "joyful," and merely a "part of life."

As the earlier theologians recognized, death can be ugly, inglorious, and joyless, and even if it is merely a part of life it is so unlike any other part that the comparison seems grotesque. Such efforts to dignify death ignore its awesomeness and finality. The Methodist theologians of the eighteenth and nineteenth centuries often seemed so intent on celebrating the promise of death that they minimized its character as penalty. But they never forgot it entirely. When Richard Watson worried that he would not be able to submit to his death, and when later Methodists told the story of Watson's dying and recalled his worries, both he and they were sustained by the theological awareness that death, as penalty, was not supposed to be simply a "part of life."[44]

Death in the Wesleyan tradition is the completion of a journey. As such, it shares the ambiguity of other completions. It terminates and fulfills. Methodists have always claimed that life lived richly and with ethical sensitivity requires a continual awareness of death, though not a morbid preoccupation with it. To speak of death is to speak of a mystery, and it is often best to speak of mysteries with paradox. In speaking of death as penalty and promise, Wesley provided a set of conceptual boundaries that precluded both despair and sentimentality. Methodists have often felt the attraction of a sentimental detour, but as long as the tradition can maintain a sensitivity to both the promise and the penalty of death, it can continue to inform our sensitivity to the dying and our acceptance of death as an enemy conquered.

# Part III

# GUIDEPOSTS

# ·5·

# Morality and Dignity

The philosophers of the eighteenth century rediscovered human dignity, and the discovery made Wesley uneasy. "How many labored panegyrics do we now read and hear on the dignity of human nature," he complained. He disliked the rhetorical celebrations of dignity because he thought that they disguised the deeper reality of human sinfulness and divine grace. He also thought that they ignored the everyday realities of human brutality and cruelty. In a world of warring nations, slave traders, torturers, and bear-baiters, it seemed absurd to talk about "the dignity of our nature."[1]

Yet when the philosopher David Hartley described human behavior as being determined by nerve vibrations and their patterned associations—and hence seemed to deny the possibility of responsible freedom—Wesley responded with a panegyric of his own: "I would fain place mankind in a fairer point of view than that writer has done," he wrote, "as I cannot believe the noblest creature in the visible world to be only a fine piece of clockwork." Wesley, the orthodox apologist for the doctrine of original sin, assumed the task of defending human nobility against the philosopher of the enlightenment.[2]

The conflict between the Wesley who disdained to praise human dignity and the Wesley who hastened to defend human nobility is only apparent. His exalting of human freedom and responsibility was, in his eyes, a defense of divine grace. And he developed an ethic of grace that drew on a wide array of doctrinal themes to provide guidance for moral decision.

Wesley never elaborated a systematic theory of ethics, detached from broader theological assertions. When he addressed ethical issues or reflected on the ethical implications of eighteenth-century science, he returned always to a doctrine of creation and a distinction between two dimensions of God's graciousness. These dimensions Wesley called—using familiar and traditional Christian language—*prevenient* and *sanctifying* grace. His combination of the themes of creation and grace shaped his ethical vocabulary and permitted him to incorporate into his moral thought two themes that have often seemed to stand apart in Christian theology: love and law. The highest ethical possibility was the life of love. But Wesley never assumed that a loving disposition alone ensured morally appropriate behavior: Christian ethics required also the structure and wisdom of rules and laws.

When later Methodists reflected on the ethics of medicine and health, they retained Wesley's appreciation for both love and law. Often they forgot the theology of grace that undergirded the ethic; sometimes they slipped into a loveless legalism; repeatedly they proclaimed an unimaginative moralism. But at its best the Methodist tradition held love and law in tension, with each checking and informing the other, and at their best Methodist theologians have recognized that only the light touch of grace keeps love from becoming sentimental indulgence and law from becoming a platform for rigid condemnation.

Wesley's vision of a human nature rendered noble by grace became a foundation in Methodism for ethics, for reflection on science and technology, and for attitudes toward such medical topics as alcoholism and drug addiction. One can see the residue of the older tradition even in current reflection by Methodist ethicists on such topics as organ transplants and truth telling in clinical settings.

In the later nineteenth and early twentieth centuries, Methodists became so intent on promoting ethical imperatives that other Protestant groups often looked askance at their activism and moralism, convinced that they had permitted the law to overwhelm the gospel. The suspicions were sometimes justified, especially when Methodists identified faithfulness with abstinence from vices. But the tradition also contained richer possibilities, and the roots of those possibilities were the older Wesleyan doctrines of creation, grace, love, and law.

## CREATION AND GRACE

Wesley's doctrine of creation was not primarily an effort to determine when and how the created order came into existence; he accepted the traditional interpretation of Genesis without question and without extended comment. Rather it was an attempt to discern the moral and religious implications of the assertion that men and women were created in the image of God and to understand the "universal restoration" when God would create "a new heaven and a new earth." Thus his doctrine of creation functioned not so much to explain the distant past as to provide a normative depiction of appropriate behavior in the present and to chart the end toward which the whole creation was groaning and travailing in its present pain. The doctrine that men and women were created in the image of God suggested ethical norms for a social order.[3]

Wesley argued that essential human nature—in its primitive integrity—embodied a natural, a political, and a moral image of God. By the natural image, Wesley meant to indicate the human capacities for understanding, will, and freedom. It was the essential nature of men and women to seek understanding, to make choices, and to exercise freedom of choice. Such a doctrine had for Wesley a clear implication for ethical standards in the practice of medicine: physicians should not, he thought, disdain the patient's understanding and consent. Wesley never elaborated a principle of "informed consent" to medical procedures, but he came close. He deplored the tendency of physicians to fill their writings "with abundance of technical terms utterly unintelligible to plain men." In Wesley's judgment, the physician bore an ethical responsibility to make medicine "plain and intelligible." Because men and women were creatures who bore the natural image of God, the physician who cared for their physical needs had also to respect their capacities of freedom and understanding.[4]

By the political image, Wesley meant to affirm that human beings rightly exercised dominion over the lower creation, the lower animal realm. But dominion implied duties, and when Wesley expounded those duties he touched on another topic that would later become a matter of concern in medical research. He thought it one of the marks of human fallenness that the lower animals were subject to unrelenting and irresponsible human cruelty. "The human shark," he observed, "torments them of his free choice." To inflict needless pain on animals seemed a clear offense against the responsibility implicit in the political image of God.[5]

By the moral image, he meant a capacity to love. The ideal of human behavior was loving concern for others. And such an ideal stood in judgment over medical practice as he saw it in eighteenth-century England. Physicians, Wesley thought, were unduly subject to motives of "honour and gain" and insufficiently willing to follow the dictate of love by identifying themselves with the suffering of their patients. Physicians had come to be viewed as "persons who were something more than human," with the result that "profit attended their employ, as well as honour," and the desire for profit overwhelmed the motive of service.[6]

He concluded that any act which destroyed or suppressed the lingering remains of the natural, political, or moral image of God contradicted human nature. Implicit in Wesley's depiction of the image of God was an ethic which prohibited the suppression of understanding, the shackling of choice, the subversion of proper dominion, and the denial of love.

The doctrine of creation thus functioned as an axiomatic foundation for ethical judgment. It elaborated the presuppositions implicit in moral demands that were binding upon every man and woman, whether Christian or not. Every ethical claim presupposes a set of dogmatic beliefs, which are usually unstated. Wesley's doctrine of creation provided a way for him to be explicit about the dogmatic beliefs underlying his own ethical judgments.

His doctrine of creation provided not only a normative depiction of the image of God but also a broader conceptual background for ethical decision. The harmony and order of the original creation offered a pattern for "a far nobler state of things," a "new creation" which would restore a natural order without pain, without destruction, without cruelty and fierceness, without wasting and violence, without sickness and death. Indeed, Wesley thought that the new creation would offer "an unmixed state of holiness and happiness, far superior to that which Adam enjoyed in paradise." But the old creation foreshadowed the new, so the description of the original created harmony offered a mythic image of the goal toward which the whole world moved. To act in accord with created human nature was also to act in anticipation of the new creation.[7]

The Fall made it impossible, of course, for men and women in their natural state to act in accord with their created nature. But Wesley supposed that every man and every woman was the beneficiary of a prevenient grace that restored in a measure each of the capacities that had marked the original image of God. By that prevenient grace, God enlightened the understanding, gently lured the will, restored liberty, and initiated a movement toward the restoration of love.

No person remained in a state of "mere nature." Every person shared a "general knowledge of good and evil" and suffered the pangs of conscience for acting "contrary to this light." Some philosophers and theologians called this capacity the "natural conscience," and Wesley was willing to accept the term. But he denied that it was natural—he thought it a supernatural gift of grace possessed by every man and woman, even "those who have not the knowledge of his written word."[8]

Because he thought that God had begun through prevenient grace to restore the divine image, Wesley believed that the norms implicit in essential human nature could even now direct moral behavior. One of his chief objections to eighteenth-century Calvinism was that the Calvinist doctrine of the bondage of the will, as he understood it, failed to furnish a foundation for good works. But he believed that prevenient grace restored the capacity for a free responsiveness to God, and that freedom entailed moral responsibility: "Indeed if man were not free, he would not be accountable either for his words, thoughts, or actions." Yet prevenient grace did more than restore liberty. Wesley believed that the "conscience" could discern the "inner law" of human nature, the divine "rule" that defined good and evil, without which the human response would be misdirected. Hence the ethical responsibility of an informed freedom became through divine grace a general human possibility.[9]

An even higher moral possibility came from the sanctifying grace vouchsafed to the faithful Christian who responded to the promptings of prevenient grace with freedom and trust. All truly good works, thought Wesley, resulted from the gift of justification and the subsequent process of sanctification, a gradual amelioration of sin and selfishness through an alteration of the temper and disposition. The doctrine of sanctification became Wesley's way of asserting that the Christian life brought about a real change in the believer, a reorientation of character and conduct. The process had ethical implications: external deeds of mercy became means by which God engendered love. "All works of mercy, whether they relate to the bodies or souls of men, such as feeding the hungry, clothing the naked, entertaining the stranger, visiting those that are in prison, or sick, or variously afflicted" formed the inner disposition of the soul.[10]

The way of love meant chiefly a love for God. Wesley criticized ethicists, like Frances Hutcheson in Scotland, who argued that true love for the neighbor could exist apart from the love of God. The biblical revelation, he thought, asserted that the love of God was the foundation of love for the neighbor and of every other virtue. When Wesley spoke of Christian perfection, he had in mind a pure love for God that issued in love for the neighbor; hence central to his ethic was the demand for purity of heart.

Wesley was interested far more in purity of intention than in the consequences of ethical activity. He admitted that perfect love could coexist with mistakes about facts and circumstances, about the goodness of actions, about the character of other persons, or about the interpretation of Scripture. Wesley's teaching about perfect love referred to the governing motive of ethical activity, not to any presumed freedom from errors of judgment or practice.[11]

An ethic of intention provides, however, little guidance about concrete ethical decisions. It stipulates only that actions issue from the motive of love. Therefore Wesley recognized that true "virtue" required more than love; it required also "truth." His insistence that loving actions be conformed to the truth could on occasion mean no more than that virtuous men and women would always appear exactly as they were. They would avoid simulation ("the seeming to be what we are not") and dissimulation ("the seeming not to be what we are"). But the requirement that loving actions be conformed to the truth could also mean that they had to be congruent with reality. For Wesley that meant they had to be in accord with the will of God. And he believed that the will of God had found expression in law.[12]

An ethic of intention, therefore, required an ethic of law. Wesley did not assume that love alone could spontaneously find its way toward the ethically appropriate deed. The quality of love in either a decision or a larger pattern of behavior determined the ethical quality of both act and life, but Wesley recognized that he provided little guidance when he simply instructed someone faced with an ethical dilemma to "act lovingly." The faithless could not act lovingly, and the faithful did not always know how to express their love appropriately.

Both the faithless and the faithful, however, could act in accordance with God's will expressed in the law. By *law* Wesley meant, first, the eternal law: "the original ideas of Truth and good which were lodged in the uncreated mind from Eternity." The law was the "supreme and unchangeable reason" standing behind visible appearances. The law in that sense was identical with the eternal reason that structured the world, and Wesley's admonition was for men and women to act in accordance with the deeper reality of things.[13]

By *law* he also meant the moral law: the model of truth and good implicit within human nature, "engraved" in the heart at creation and "reinscribed" after the Fall. The moral law was identical with the deeper structure of human nature, which both the "heathen" and the faithful could discern as a rule for conscience. Thus Wesley did not hesitate to condemn certain practices as inconsistent with human nature. He condemned African slavery not only because of its cruelty but also because it contradicted human nature by treating men and women as if they had no liberty: "Give liberty to whom liberty is due, that is, to every child of man, to every partaker of human nature." Slavery also contradicted the true nature of the slaveholder: to be a human being, he thought, was to share a capacity for compassion and sympathy. Because slavery so obviously dampened that capacity, it stood condemned by the moral law that lay deep within human nature.[14]

By *law* Wesley meant also the written moral law in Scripture, published in the Old and New Testaments and bringing to light the hidden depths of the law engraved in human nature. Wesley did not believe that Christ had abolished the moral law. He had provided a means of salvation even for Christians unable to fulfill the law, but he did not destroy it: "There is no contrariety at all between the law and the gospel; . . . there is no need for the law to pass away, in order to the establishing of the gospel."[15]

Among Wesley's best-known series of sermons were his discourses "Upon Our Lord's Sermon on the Mount," in which he tried to provide "a general view of the whole" of Christianity. The chief aim of the sermons was to depict the Christian way as the way of love, and to argue that the gospel showed Christians not simply "how to be" but also "what to do." Wesley found in the ethical injunctions of the Sermon on the Mount a realistic prescription for Christian piety and moral behavior. Hence he could also argue that the "revealed law of God," with its stipulation of mercy as a higher way, condemned any practice, such as slavery, that was "utterly inconsistent with mercy."[16]

By *law*, finally, Wesley meant civil law, the regulations of king and parliament specifying what was "due" unto Caesar. Wesley was more than willing to render Caesar his due. He was, in politics, a consistent Tory who found in the Bible the plain command that Christians were not to "speak evil of the ruler." The chief duty of the Christian minister who spoke on political topics was therefore to refute any aspersions against "men in public offices."[17]

Nevertheless, the civil law stood subject always to the eternal and moral law. Wesley recognized that slavery was "authorized by law," but he refused to accept legal custom as a ground for moral acceptability. "Can law, human law, change the nature of things? Can it turn darkness into light, or evil into good? By no means. Notwithstanding ten thousand laws, right is right, and wrong is wrong, still. There must still remain an essential difference between justice and injustice, cruelty and mercy."[18]

In addition to distinguishing the several dimensions of the law, Wesley also formulated more specific rules to govern the behavior of his Methodists. When he organized his "societies," he stipulated that the members had to obey three general rules. First, they were to do no harm. They were not to fight, quarrel, brawl, buy and sell distilled liquors, practice usury, speak uncharitably, wear costly apparel, or enjoy frivolous diversions. Second, they were to do good. They were to feed the hungry, clothe the naked, visit the sick, help the imprisoned, assist other Christians in business and trade, and stand ready always with words of instruction and exhortation. Third, they were to attend upon the ordinances of God: public worship, private prayer, fasting, and the study of Scripture. They were to remain subject, in all that they did, to rules that lent themselves to precise specification and definition.[19]

For Wesley, then, law and love never stood in tension. He remained confident that they would always cohere. But such a confidence would not always mark the Methodist tradition.

## FROM RULES TO PERSONS

Methodists never relinquished their appreciation for laws and rules in moral reflection, but they became increasingly sensitive to possible conflicts between what the law might demand and what love might require. To relate the history of ethical reflection within the Methodist tradition is to return repeatedly to efforts at balancing the demands of love and law. An understanding of that history illumines certain persistent themes in Methodist ethical reflection on topics of medicine and health.

Early Methodist theologians could hardly ignore the moral philosophers of the eighteenth century who tried to free ethics from theological encumbrances. Methodists resisted the innovation but nevertheless drew on the ideas and images of the innovators. A good example is Richard Watson, who included in his *Theological Institutes* in 1823 a separate section on the "morals of Christianity," thus establishing a pattern for later nineteenth-century Methodist theological textbooks.

Watson criticized the presumption of the new "moral philosophers"—Frances Hutcheson, Samuel Clarke, William Wollaston—whom he accused of treating ethics as a "separate science" and distracting attention from the "revealed law of God." Yet he also drew heavily on their ethical theories. Before long, Methodists were publishing their own textbooks in moral philosophy.[20]

The Methodist moral philosophers relied on the revealed law, but they also relied on philosophical theories, especially those of Samuel Clarke, an eighteenth-century Anglican divine who had defined moral rectitude as conformity to the "eternal and necessary fitness of things." Like Clarke, they tried to discern fitting behavior by observing the "relations" which structured human society. Because human beings existed always in relation to God, to other human beings (as husbands or wives, parents or children, masters or servants), and to themselves, they stood under the duties imposed by each relation. The task of the moral philosophers was to specify the appropriate duties, a task for which they found guidance in both the scriptural law and the law of love.[21]

The idea of relations provided an alternative to a utilitarian moral scheme that determined the quality of moral actions by asking whether they promoted the greatest good of the greatest number. To the Methodist moral philosophers, it seemed clear that future consequences were always beyond precise calculation, and that, in any event, the utilitarians offered no criterion to determine what the "greatest good" in any given case might be. The Methodists believed that actions were right insofar as they conformed to the divine moral law, which required both purity of intention and behavior appropriate to the existing pattern of relations to God, neighbor, and self. The "right" was conformity to a law.[22]

The Methodist moral philosophers dealt explicitly with medicine and health only when they explicated the third set of relations—our relations to ourselves—and outlined the "duties to ourselves" that such relations seemed to require. It appeared obvious to them that certain laws—including the "law of our physical being"—determined our duties to ourselves and that obedience to such laws required proper regard to diet, the avoidance of overeating and improper drinking, healthy exercise, and reasonable apparel designed for health and comfort. Any unhealthy apparel—like tight corsets—represented a transgression of the law. By the same law of duty to ourselves, suicide stood condemned.[23]

A conception of ethical behavior as conformity to specifiable laws remained popular among Methodist theologians throughout the early nineteenth century. But by the time William Burt Pope in England published his *Compendium of Christian Theology* in 1875, Methodists were tiring of the relentless accent on law. Pope still described Christian virtue as obedience to the laws of God, but he observed that when "love" interpreted the laws, it could often find a "deeper meaning" than a surface reading might suggest.

"The Christian revelation," he wrote, "is comparatively indifferent to legal codes and formal enactments. It does not dwell so much on the enforcement of specific obligations as on the vigorous maintenance of the principle of charity." The internal law of love enabled the Christian to exercise "a peculiar freedom and irregularity" even while remaining obedient to external laws. Love was the "casuist" which presided over such anomalies in ethics as conflicting laws and the collision of duties.[24]

Without abandoning the theme of law, Methodist writers in the late nineteenth century turned their attention from rules and obedience to "character" and "personality." The aim of ethics seemed increasingly to be the formation of character and of respect for personality. The English editor W. L. Watkinson, for example, urged Methodists to think of ethics as a search for beauty of character: "We are apt to be content with a hard propriety of conduct which falls far short of poetry. We fulfill the commandments of God, discharge the duties of life, exemplify the virtues, without reaching the mark that is known as beauty."[25] The goal of these ethicists was the creation of persons who would act rightly without having to reflect about it. The American theologian John Tigert insisted that "the real business of life, beside which there is none other worthy of mention, is the formation of such a sensitive moral nature that the good shall be uniformly and spontaneously accepted, and the evil as uniformly and spontaneously rejected." The ideal of character provided a new way of talking about the older doctrine of sanctification, and it also suggested that ethical sensitivity required far more than a plodding conformity to laws and rules.[26]

The English Methodist Hugh Price Hughes could therefore proclaim in 1889 that "we are Christian just so far as the Love of God has been reproduced in us; just so far as we love one another in the very same way in which God, that is Christ, loves us." A few Methodists in the late nineteenth century began to move beyond a preoccupation with rules and laws and to speak simply of the "law of love." The appeal to the law of love became a rallying cry, for instance, among the English Methodists who carried Hughes's "gospel of health" into the urban slums.[27]

Hughes argued that the law of love required a concern for the physical health of the poor. His disciples established urban settlement houses to minister to both physical and spiritual needs. In the Bermondsey settlement which they founded in London in 1891, for example, they not only provided education and recreation but also secured the help of medical students to offer free medical care. They saw themselves as transcending the narrow legalism of an earlier era—which had often condemned the poor for vices and transgressions. They would try to be of service to the miserable rather than condemning them for their misery.[28]

"The Christian ethic is an ethic of love," wrote the Methodist theologian Albert Knudson in 1943, "and it is such because the Christian world is a personal world and a personal world is a social world." In connecting the ethic of love to the theme of personality, Knudson was expressing a popular point of view among Methodists in the first half of the twentieth century. Among liberal Methodist theologians, at any rate, the chief criterion for moral judgment often became respect for personality.[29]

This was especially true among the influential party of American Methodists who looked for guidance to a philosophical theologian at Boston University named Borden Parker Bowne. Bowne's accent on the "supreme significance of the moral personality" would deeply inform Methodist ethical reflection after he became the founder of a theological tradition known as personalism, the view that the world of space and time was the expression of an underlying personal life, and that God as the Supreme Person ensured the "inviolable sacredness" of moral persons who had an "absolute value" in themselves.[30]

Subsequent Methodist ethicists modified Bowne's emphasis on the sacredness of personality. Georgia Harkness observed in her *Christian Ethics* in 1957, for example, that Jesus had never spoken of the "intrinsic worth of personality." But she added that Jesus had declared the "supreme worth of every person to God." This concept of the sacredness of the person as a child of God remained, in one form or another, an honored theme in Methodist ethical reflection. The "guidelines for strategy" in social action published by American Methodists in 1962 expressed a consensus in the tradition when, in their outline of the principles of Christian ethics, they announced that "the first principle is the dignity and worth of the human person as a child of God."[31]

When Methodists seek warrants for their positions on questions of medicine and health, they return often to the concept of the inviolability of the person. Throughout the 1970s and 1980s, delegates to the General Conference of the United Methodist Church could encourage support for mental health programs on the grounds that the Bible exhibited a concern for the "development of the whole person." They could call for a "pediatric bill of rights" because they believed that "every child . . . has the right to be regarded as a person" and receive "rights as a person." They supported additional aid from governments for the health care of children because they thought that "we must nurture and protect their rights as persons created by God and in his image." The notion of the inviolability of the person has thus become a standard modern restatement of Wesley's doctrine of the *imago dei.*[32]

Whereas Wesley supplemented his doctrine of the image of God with a detailed elaboration of the theme of law, twentieth-century Methodists have often been inclined to contrast concern for persons and conformity to codes. The changing Methodist attitudes toward alcohol and alcoholism illustrate the movement from rules to persons. Few religious traditions have been more closely identified with opposition to alcohol than the Methodists, especially in England and America. To be sure, not all Methodists share that antagonism: Methodists in Germany found the temperance movement puzzling, while Methodists in America embraced it. For some, abstinence from alcohol became a holy cause. In 1908 the delegates to one General Conference in America could declare that "the Methodist Episcopal Church is a temperance society."[33]

Writing in a century when England drunkenly staggered to work in the mornings, Wesley had scorned drunkenness. He thought it a flouting of human nature—and hence of the moral law—when the drunkard discarded reason and assumed the demeanor of beasts and demons. "The drunkard is a public enemy," he said. The drunkard crucified Christ anew by denying his power and love; rebelled against king and country; rebelled even against God. Yet Wesley distinguished between the sinner and the sin: "I beseech you, brethren, by the mercies of God, do not despise poor drunkards! Have compassion on them! Be instant with them in season and out of season! Let not shame, or fear of men, prevent you pulling these brands out of the burning."[34]

He recognized that the abuse of distilled liquors in eighteenth-century England had created social suffering on an immense scale. Wesley therefore urged a legal ban on distilling, and he made the members of his United Societies promise that they would forswear both drunkenness and "buying or selling spirituous liquors, or drinking them, unless in cases of extreme necessity," by which he meant medical necessity rather than inordinate thirst. Methodists could "taste no spirituous liquor, no dram of any kind, unless prescribed by a physician." In his *Primitive Physick* he described "spirituous liquors" as "slow poison." Thus he dealt with the problem through legal proscription. Drunkenness was wrong because it flouted a law (and brought misery). Drunkenness could be fought by the promulgation of a law, whether by Parliament or by Wesley himself.[35]

Despite his suspicion of distillers and distilled drinks, he had no objection to milder fermented alcohol. He drank ale and brewed it in his home, and in his medical guide he recommended small beer as a healthy ingredient in a plain diet. He frequently drank a glass of wine, and he recommended the same to the readers of his medical treatises: "I cannot but think, if your wine is good in kind, suited to your constitution, and taken in small quantities, it is full as wholesome as any liquor in the world, except water." He left off the wine for two years when a doctor suggested that abstinence might improve his health, but he resumed his custom when some of his disciples and critics concluded that he had made abstention "a point of conscience." Wesley warned against the abuse of both wine and ale, but he did not make them the objects of legal proscription. He considered wine to be "one of the noblest cordials in nature."[36]

The nineteenth-century temperance movement therefore met with a mixed response from English Methodists. It was customary among Methodists in England to drink home-brewed beer at circuit dinners and Sunday School festivals, and those convivial folk felt offended by temperance reformers. In

1841, the Wesleyan Methodist Church forbade the members of any chapel to open the buildings for temperance meetings. It also forbade the use of unfermented grape juice in place of wine in the sacrament, and it placed restrictions on Methodist preachers who wanted to advocate "teetotalism" among the faithful. Only among the Primitive Methodists who had separated from the main body in 1812 did temperance societies find a welcome.[37]

Methodists in America proved equally resistant to the demand for abstinence. They prohibited their members from drinking or retailing spirituous liquors, but the General Conference in 1812 refused to approve a motion that "no stationed or local preacher shall retail spirituous liquors without forfeiting his ministerial character among us." For years they squabbled over the issue in their conference sessions. Could members of Methodist societies distill spirits? Could they buy and sell?

The advocates of temperance insisted that the use of ardent spirits was inconsistent with happiness and usefulness; that spirituous alcohol was poisonous; that the Bible forbade drunkenness; that no safe line could be drawn between the moderate and the immoderate use of alcohol. But not until 1848, after the denomination had divided over the issue of slavery, did the northern Methodists come out in favor of total abstinence. The cause would remain suspect for years in the South.[38]

Among Methodists in the northern United States, the drive for temperance prospered, and the denomination maintained strict rules against offenders. By 1864 the northerners were recommending that only the pure juice of the grape be used even in the celebration of the Lord's Supper. Numberless Methodists eventually began to conceive of abstinence from the consumption of alcohol not as simply a matter of health but as a religious obligation, indeed as the primary symbol of one's commitment as a Christian, and although conservatives, especially in the South, resisted the temperance movement, the Methodists soon cast their lot wholeheartedly with the prohibitionists.[39]

Despite the appearance among Methodist ethicists of a disinclination to rely on rules and laws, the Methodist churches in the late nineteenth century continued to pass and enforce a host of regulations about whiskey, wine, and beer. The grounds for opposition to alcohol occasionally changed. In the late nineteenth century, both in England and America, the refrain was that abstinence would save society from grievous evils; the champions of the social gospel tended to be advocates of the temperance movement. The demand for abstinence helped as well to shape the new ideal of character. But Methodists could also reply to inquiries by simply appealing to the laws of the church: "We refer to our General Rule on this subject."[40]

The tension between an ethic of law and a personalist ethic in the temperance movement appeared explicitly in the reformist activities of the Woman's Christian Temperance Union (W.C.T.U.), founded in 1874 and destined to lead in the struggle against alcohol. Frances E. Willard, a Methodist laywoman who became the most powerful figure in the organization, insisted, in writing the Declaration of Principles, that temperance reform was part of a larger concern for human personality. She therefore connected the topic of alcohol abuse with other social problems: a living wage, an eight-hour day, equality between men and women, and courts of conciliation and arbitration. And she trusted mainly in the power of education: she wanted schools to adopt courses on the nature and effects of alcohol, and many of them did.[41]

When the Anti-Saloon League of America came into existence in 1895, its purpose to settle the issue with the aid of politicians and legislation, the W.C.T.U. gave the new prohibitionist organization its support, but Willard felt ambivalent about the political coercion. She preferred argument, education, and persuasion, and she thought that they would be more effective in the long run. At the time, her hesitations seemed timid and old-fashioned; the prohibitionists abandoned her preference for study and education and placed their trust in other measures. The emphasis on education about alcohol reemerged only a couple of decades after the passage of the Eighteenth Amendment, though "by that time the word *alcohol* had changed to *alcoholism*."[42]

As early as 1872, a few Methodists were writing of alcoholism as a disease and calling for treatment centers, but not until after the Second World War did such a conception of the problem attract widespread support. During the 1950s, the *Methodist Message*, the journal of the church in Southeast Asia, announced that a new approach had begun to exert considerable influence on the Methodist strategy of temperance education: "It has arisen," the journal explained, "out of a concern for the alcoholic." In 1956 the General Conference of the Methodist Church in America called on its members to "seek to understand the causes of alcoholism and drug addiction, and to give help to their victims in a healing and redemptive ministry and fellowship."[43]

The new strategy reflected the changing conceptions of alcoholism among physicians and scientists, and also the changing attitudes toward alcohol in the social groups from which Methodists drew members. By the 1960s, one poll could show that 65 percent of Methodists in the United States supported total abstinence from alcoholic beverages; another poll, that 61 percent of Methodists refused to abstain. But in any case, they had begun to consider alcoholism a signal not so much of rules broken as of bodies and spirits diseased. By 1980, Methodists were urging that the health system accept alcoholism as a medical, social, and behavioral problem, and treat the alcoholic with the same attention and consideration given any other patient.[44]

The tendency to think of alcoholism as a disease coincided with the inclination to appeal to "personality" as the chief criterion of ethical judgment. In 1940, even before the newer understanding of alcoholism attracted popular support, a Methodist General Conference appealed to the concept of personality as the motive for abstinence: "The teaching of Christ emphasizes as one of its basic principles the sacredness of each human personality. Anything which blights personality is fundamentally opposed to the Gospel of Christ. Since alcohol by its very nature harms personality, we stand for the Christian principle of total abstinence."[45]

The same moral reasoning reappeared in 1976 as an expression of "deep concern" for persons who are dependent on alcohol and drugs: "The church can offer a religious and moral heritage which views each individual as a person of infinite worth and significance, sees meaning and purpose in all of life, supports the individual and the society in the quest for wholeness and fulfillment, and seeks healing for the afflicted and liberty for the oppressed."[46] By 1972, Methodists in America were resuming the older debates about alcohol, and after protracted controversy the General Conference of the United Methodist Church decided to broaden the context for interpreting its traditional opposition to the use of alcohol. It asserted its "long-standing conviction" that the "choice to abstain from alcohol" was a "faithful witness to God's liberating and redeeming love for persons." But by 1976 it also warned against the spirit of legalistic condemnation: "Christian love in human relationships is primary, thereby making abstinence an instrument of love and always subject to the requirements of love. Persons who practice abstinence should avoid attitudes of self-righteousness which express moral superiority and condemnatory attitudes toward those who do not abstain."[47]

By 1976, the transition from an ethic of rules to a personalistic ethic, along with parallel transitions in scientific research and cultural mores, had reshaped attitudes toward alcohol among Methodists. The issue continued to mark lines of division within the tradition, with some conservatives deeply upset at what they perceived to be a movement away from earlier certainties. But few Methodists referred any longer simply to the "general rules," and declining numbers continued to think of alcoholism simply as a sign of moral failure.

The understanding of alcoholism as a medical problem found expression in a new strategy for counseling alcoholics and their families. In 1956, the pastoral theologian Howard J. Clinebell, Jr., published the first edition of his guidebook on *Understanding and Counseling the Alcoholic*. Drawing on medical and scientific research, he urged ministers to recognize that alcoholism was a disease symptomatic of deeper psychological, physiological, social, and religious disorders. His conclusion was that moralistic condemnation of alcoholics tended to diminish the possibilities of cure because it increased feelings of guilt and unworthiness, pushing the suffering alcoholic toward a spiral of hidden despair that made cure more difficult. Only when alcoholics were encouraged to view their condition as a sickness, he argued, would they seek the help they must have in order to recover, obtain medical treatment, and achieve a resynthesis of their lives without alcohol. The religious counselor who worked with alcoholics needed to help them understand that they needed help. Such a program of counseling would entail close cooperation with physicians as well as a sensitivity to deeper religious needs.[48]

Clinebell's guide for counselors, which has been popular among Methodist ministers, reflected both a personalist ethic and the repudiation of an older legalism. Yet Clinebell recognized that it could be useful for alcoholics to join together in sympathetic but demanding groups which would insist that their members admit their "wrongs," seek forgiveness from persons they had harmed, and continually take personal inventory so that when they wronged others they would promptly acknowledge it. In brief, he proposed something of the balance of law and love that had historically marked the Methodist tradition. He thus anticipated later debates among Methodist ethicists who would appeal to both love and law when they strove to protect the sanctity of persons threatened by dilemmas of modern medicine.[49]

In their attitudes toward science and technology, including medical science and medical technology, Methodists have revealed a similar preoccupation with the sanctity of persons. Wesley believed that it was "our duty to contemplate what [God] has wrought, and to understand as much of it as we are able."[50] Such an understanding required attentiveness to the eighteenth-century field of "natural philosophy," and Wesley compiled and edited a five-volume *Compendium of Natural Philosophy* in which he surveyed the field in hopes of illustrating its usefulness for the Christian. He had high praise for some of the patriarchs of modern science—Francis Bacon, William Harvey, and the members of the Royal Society—and he celebrated their studies of blood circulation and blood transfusions, magnetism and microscopes, barometers and air pumps.

Wesley also celebrated the medical discoveries of the physicians:

> It cannot be denied that physicians have signally improved this branch of philosophy, as they have continual opportunities of making new discoveries in the human body. In diseases themselves, the wonderful wisdom of the Author of nature appears; and by means of them many hidden recesses of the human frame are unexpectedly discovered. The powers of medicines also, variously exerting themselves, lay open many secrets of nature.[51]

Such praise of the sciences issued from Wesley's confidence that "religion and reason go hand in hand." He considered it "a fundamental principle with us, that to renounce reason is to renounce religion."[52]

Yet Wesley was also intent on locating the limits of natural philosophy, and he felt that its most impenetrable limit was its inability fully to grasp either God or the human being. Wesley was convinced that we knew little about the human spirit. "What is spirit?" he asked. Where is it lodged? In the pineal gland? In the brain? In any single part of the body? "Or, is it (if anyone can understand those terms) all in all, and all in every part?" The understanding both of God and of spirit seemed to elude scientific inquiry. "In the tracing of this we can neither depend upon reason nor experiment." Hence Wesley advised his readers to turn to the Scripture, to walk in the "good old paths." Natural philosophy fell into pretension when it presumed to explain the deepest mysteries of human nature.[53]

Wesley's attitudes toward science endured among early nineteenth-century Methodist theologians. It became a commonplace among them that the findings of natural philosophers enabled them to look up "through nature's works to nature's God."[54] The only problem was to ensure the proper conduct of scientific investigation. The theologians felt ready to support science as long as it did not presume to be metaphysics or ethics. "Science, in general and in particular," wrote an American Methodist in 1855, "is merely accurate knowledge, systematically deduced from established principles and observed facts, by the mind acting according to its inherent powers and appointed laws." It should not be restricted by any religious authority, he said, but he also implied that it should not be treated as a religious or ethical authority.[55]

Methodists worried about science partly because they thought themselves obliged to insist on the sacredness of persons. When Charles Darwin published his *Origin of Species* in 1859, the primary issue for Methodists was the sanctity of the personality. In 1871, James H. Rigg, the principal of the Methodists' Westminster Training Institution in London, delivered to the Christian Evidence Society an address that received widespread

attention within English Methodism. Rigg described himself as a respectful student and admirer of Darwin's scientific accomplishment, but he
inserted a reservation: "To me it appears that the sense of personality is an
altogether new and original fact, one which cannot be conceived as developed out of any pre-existing phenomena or conditions."[56]

This was the enduring Methodist theme. W. H. Dallinger, editor of the
English *Wesleyan Methodist Magazine*, accepted most of the Darwinian
hypothesis, but he continued to affirm that the development of human beings from lower forms was "nowhere indicated in nature," and he insisted
that even if men and women, as physical creatures, did develop from lower
forms, "the moral and spiritual properties of [the] personality" had surely
been imparted directly by God. Dallinger's Fernley Lecture in 1887 at
Wesley College in Sheffield announced his agreement with the essentials of
the Darwinian hypothesis, but he concluded his lecture by assuring his
listeners that Darwinism left "unaltered our conviction of the dignity and
majesty" of human beings. In 1875 a contributor to the *Wesleyan Methodist
Magazine* delineated the precise limits of Methodist acceptance of scientific
theory: "At the very vestibule of man's moral nature we take our stand, and
affirm that the temple is sacred."[57]

By the end of the nineteenth century, Methodist theologians increasingly
made peace with Darwin and incorporated his theories into new arguments for purpose and order in nature. They could accept his conclusions
because they discovered ways to make them compatible with their traditional solicitude for the sacredness of the personality. The personalist Borden Bowne could argue, for instance, that the creation of personality was
obviously the apex of evolutionary development. Properly interpreted,
evolutionary theory coincided with the traditional Christian insistence on
the uniqueness of persons.[58]

After the two world wars of the twentieth century, and the emergence of
a neoorthodox theology that called into question those theological impulses
toward anthropocentrism, the theologians became more circumspect in
their language about human dignity. They spoke far more frequently of
human limits. But when they worried about science and technology, they
retained the time-honored Wesleyan solicitude for the sanctity of persons.

An American General Conference meeting in 1968, for example, took
note of new biomedical technologies, such as organ transplants and the
control of genetic defects. The conference observed that they both offered
rich potential for enhancing health and created renewed threats to traditional images of human nature and the values those images had preserved.[59]
In its concern for the effect of scientific and technological change on human

dignity, the conference stood in continuity with the nineteenth-century theologians who insisted in their own way on bringing ethical judgments to bear on scientific innovations.

The ethicist J. Robert Nelson, writing in 1980, reminded Methodists that science was still "a worrisome factor for people of faith," not because of any presumed threat to biblical literalism but because of a deeper issue: "What are the scientific world view and technological growth doing to the conception of human value and individual identity?" Most Methodist theologians today regret the tone and substance of the nineteenth-century Methodist criticisms of evolutionary theory, but it is useful to recall that the wariness arose not simply from obscurantism but also from an ethical regard for the sacredness of persons. Although Methodist theologians no longer oppose evolutionary theories of human origins, they do continue to insist that a concern for the sanctity of persons must inform scientific and medical research.[60]

It is easy to see the continuity between Wesley's ethic of creation and grace and the later Methodist preoccupation with the sanctity of persons. Wesley drew conclusions about the ethics of medicine from his doctrines of the image of God and sanctification. The later Methodist language about the sacredness of the personality represented an extension and adaptation of the older Wesleyan doctrines.

It is also easy to see the continuity between Wesley's accent on the law of love and the later Methodist love ethic. But whereas Wesley felt comfortable laying out the rules through which love expressed itself, later Methodists have been more impressed by the tension between love and law. Wesley's rules, some of them petty, have seemed ill-fitted to guide decisions about the ambiguous dilemmas in such a complicated sphere as medicine. Yet appeals to people to love one another and to show "respect for personality" can seem to be vague and formless ethical incantations. Hence much of the debate among twentieth-century Methodist ethicists has represented a struggle to maintain a balance between love and law. And the discussion has often turned on questions of medical ethics.

## LOVE AND LAW REVISITED

One need only encounter the difficult questions of medical ethics to discover the limits of the simple injunction to love. Consider, for example, the advances in medical technology that make it possible for a healthy person to donate organs to someone in need of them. Clearly such a gift can be a profound expression of love. But the morally sensitive physician who invites or solicits such a donation must also ask whether such an invitation is an appropriate gesture of love toward the donor. The physician must balance the good of the donor's bodily integrity against the good of the patient's probable recovery, with whatever ambiguities might cloud the prospect of recovery. It seems less than satisfactory to tell the conscientious physician to act lovingly. The physician is seeking to discern what constitutes the loving act.

Or consider the physician who must determine which patients will receive kidney dialysis when the procedure cannot be made available to everyone who needs it. To advise the physician to make the decision lovingly is hardly to participate in a serious discussion about the applicability or usefulness of criteria of selection. Or consider even the more familiar question of whether the physician should disclose to patients the full truth about their condition and their treatment, even if disclosure might diminish the possibilities of recovery. How does love discern the appropriate balance between the possibly conflicting values of truthfulness and the recovery of health?

The Methodist tradition has no fixed solutions for such ethical dilemmas. But the dilemmas have helped to prompt a second look at the relationship between love and law as an ethical problem.

On one point, the theologians seem to have reached a consensus. Like the Methodist moral philosophers of the early nineteenth century, they agree about the inadequacy of a simple utilitarian solution to ethical problems in medicine. The mere probability that a course of action—say, medical experimentation on human subjects—would produce clear benefits for future generations provides no warrant for proceeding with the experiment. "There must be a determination," writes Paul Ramsey, "of the rightness or wrongness of the action and not only of the good to be obtained in medical care or from medical investigation." Such a determination entails, at the least, "the requirement of a reasonably free and adequately informed consent."[61]

Clinton Gardner, an ethicist at Emory University, grounds such a requirement in the "primacy of the subject as a person," thus appealing to the criteria of love for the neighbor and the sanctity of persons. Whatever its grounding, the requirement of consent stands in tension with the simple utilitarian judgment that experimental research must continue for the sake of a greater social good. In the absence of consent, say these ethicists, the research should not continue, despite its promise of social benefit.[62]

In writing of the need for informed consent on the part of subjects in medical experimentation, the theologians are advancing a principle to guide moral reflection. Like Wesley, who urged physicians to avoid mystifying language on the grounds that respect for the natural image of God in the creature entailed the obligation to respect human liberty and understanding, the ethicists who argue for informed consent are appealing to a moral generalization. However they might interpret the logical status of the generalization, they are advancing a principle that functions much in the same way that formulations of the moral law functioned for Wesley. And they are therefore assuming that a lawlike principle informs and guides the loving intention.

Methodist theologians today rarely write about the "eternal law" or the "moral law" in the same way Wesley did. Most would agree with the judgment of Bruce Birch and Larry Rasmussen:

> The touchstone for Israel's morality and that of the early church is always the faith-experience of God. All the elements used in determining which behavior is most fitting in a given set of circumstances take their form and function from this faith relationship. This means, to cite but one example, that rules, principles and other norms in the decision making process are viewed as expressive of underlying relationships, indicating their kind, quality, and content. The rules, principles and other norms take their authority from the defining relationships, not the reverse.[63]

Even when Methodist theologians speak of laws or principles as moral generalizations that derive their authority from the commitments and responses of a community of faith, most of them do not share Wesley's confidence that one can isolate appropriate rules that will embody Christian love in almost every situation. Insofar as they remain in continuity with the tradition, though, they are sensitive to the function of principles and rules as guidelines in ethical reflection.

An example of the continuity is to be found in the history of Methodist comment on the issue of truth telling, an issue of obvious relevance for decisions about the complete disclosure of information in medical practice. Wesley had no doubt about the proper course of action for the Christian: "Nothing but truth is heard from his mouth." Christian veracity was an obedience to the express command of God in Ephesians 4:25: "Putting away all lying, speak every man truth to his neighbor." He recognized that numerous Christian writers had justified what he called "officious lies, those that are spoken with a design to do good." But Wesley appealed to Romans 3:7–8: "If the truth of God hath more abounded through my lie unto his glory, why am I yet judged as a sinner?" He concluded that "the good effect of a lie is no excuse for it." The prohibition against falsehood was absolute, and Wesley found no absurdity in "that saying of the ancient father, 'I would not tell a wilful lie, to save the souls of the whole world.'" Hence he interpreted the question of veracity primarily as a matter of obedience or disobedience to a binding law. Whatever the consequences, he thought, the truth must be told.[64]

In the middle of the nineteenth century, Methodist moralists still upheld the sanctity of truth, but they appealed to a different understanding of law and they began to take note of exceptions to the rule. The moral philosopher R. H. Rivers, for example, defined moral truth as "the conformity of our words to our opinions" and insisted that the obligation to be morally truthful was so binding that the conscientious person would make "an investigation as thorough as possible . . . before risking a statement." He found a warrant for his position in the popular philosophical theory of "relations": "The relations established by God between man and man—relations of mutual dependence and reciprocity—indicate most clearly that we are under obligation to tell the truth."[65] Against the claim of Archdeacon William Paley that a falsehood was no lie when it failed to deceive or when it deceived a person who had no right to know the truth, Rivers responded by insisting that motives to deceive were always base. He interpreted the requirement of veracity primarily as a matter of conformity to a fixed rule which governed purity of motive. But he recognized permissible exceptions: deception might be justified, he acknowledged, in order to save innocent life.[66]

By the early twentieth century, the personalist theologian Albert Knudson grounded the duty of truthfulness on the argument that truth telling was necessary to sustain the mutual confidence undergirding social welfare and personal growth. The assertion that one should tell the truth was a rule implied in the larger values of mutuality and fulfillment. Hence the larger values set limits to the duty of truthfulness. "We feel no obligation," he wrote, "to tell the truth to a person who is seriously ill if doing so would imperil or lessen his chances of recovery." In Knudson's construal of the problem, a concern for pure motives and proper conformity to rules faded before the larger need to maintain the values of trust and mutuality as indispensable conditions for personal growth. Hence he treated the principle of truth telling as instrumental in the preservation of higher principles, and he felt free to subordinate the lower principle to the higher ones.[67]

James Laney's "Ethics and Death" (1969) illustrated a growing tendency among Methodists to avoid a formalistic legalism and to frame the question of truth telling in the light of responsibility to the patient rather than of obedience to a law or conformity to a principle. The issue, he said, was "settled neither by an appeal to the patient's right to the truth in some general sense, nor derived from one's universal obligation to veracity in a Kantian sense." According to Laney, the communication of "truth" within a relationship should be distinguished from the utterance of cold, objective facts. Someone making a decision about truth telling had to consider the relationship of the patient to the truth-teller; the trust and confidence between them; the probable medical consequences of candor; the subtle danger that evasion could establish an atmosphere of subterfuge which might taint beneficial supporting relationships; the necessity not to abandon the patient; the patient's need for honest and sustaining care; the patient's need to come to terms with an impending death within a community of loving friends; and the dangers of simply bludgeoning the patient with truth, however well-intentioned. Laney was concerned about "truth responsibly uttered," and his concern led to a critical stance toward a facile reliance on general principles.[68]

Yet Laney also relied throughout his article on both explicit and implicit moral generalizations: One should value human life; one should attend to any possibility of beneficial recovery and act so as not to preclude it; one should never abandon the dying; one should care about the sensibilities and feelings of persons. Rather than addressing a presumed conflict between responsibility to principles and responsibility to persons, his argument took account of conflicts among ethical principles. Yet he employed those principles within a moral discourse intended to form and discipline love and enhance love's awareness of ethical complexity.

Ethicists within modern Methodism do not agree about the function and status of general ethical principles. Some use moral generalizations to determine the appropriate ends of moral conduct; others use them to reflect on the appropriate means of achieving ends. Some consider principles to be prescriptive. They argue that Christian moral principles prescribe right conduct for Christians. Others consider them to be only illuminative. They believe that principles help to enrich moral discourse and form moral vision, but without defining in advance how one should respond in every situation. In either case, they reflect a discernible style of ethical argumentation, characterized by the effort to balance love and law, disposition and rule. Such a style of argument distantly echoes some of Wesley's cherished theological assumptions.[69]

Following from his doctrine of the creation of man and woman in the image of God, Wesley could assume that certain moral claims had their grounds in the requirements of human nature and did not depend exclusively on special revelation for their force and obligation. Because of his doctrine of prevenient grace, he could appeal to philosophical and common-sense principles without having to assume either that they were so tainted by original sin as to be useless or that the persons to whom he addressed them were so trapped within original sin as to be closed to moral argument. Because of his conviction that grace did not render law otiose, he could assume the usefulness of laws and rules not only to restrain the sinful and drive them to Christ but also to guide moral decisions within the community of faith. And because he thought of the Christian way as the way of love, he assumed that ethical sensitivity required far more than formal obedience to rules and commandments.

The tradition has not always shared Wesley's confidence in the capacity of the law to embody the imperatives of love. Methodists have, in fact, often wavered between a legalism that identified love with conformity to rules and an ethic of pure intention that assumed the intrinsic wisdom of love. At their best, however, they have avoided both legalism and sentimentalism. In any case, they have consistently, insofar as they remained within the boundaries of the tradition, explored ethical dilemmas by wrestling with the tensions and harmonies between love and law.

# ·6·

# Passages and Sexuality

In his *Explanatory Notes Upon the New Testament*, John Wesley explained that Jesus had "passed through and sanctified every stage of human life," except for old age. Jesus had been an infant, and then a child, and then an adult.[1] Like the Apostle Paul, Wesley found it useful to refer to those stages of human life when he tried to explain the gospel. He described the Christian journey from sin to salvation with metaphors taken from the everyday passages of common experience: birth, the awakening of the senses, growth, maturity, and death. He thought of Christians as being babes in Christ or "grown up to the measure of the stature of Christ."[2]

Wesley was intent on discerning how the larger Christian journey altered our understanding of the natural passages through which every person proceeds as a biological, sexual, and social creature. He also wanted to know how those natural passages affected the course of the Christian journey.

He had his own ideas, for example, about how the experience of being a child altered one's religious propensities, or about what might be expected from older Christians. He recognized that each stage of life had its distinctive tasks: childhood was a time for disciplined growth; adulthood was a time for work and worship; old age was a period in which the saintly bore a special authority. He thought, too, that each stage had its special temptations: childhood was a time of self-will; adulthood introduced new forms of sinfulness; old age could bring pride, or unwise indulgence for oneself or others.[3]

The stresses of the natural passages, left unchecked, could hinder progress in the larger Christian journey. A recurring theme in Wesley's discussions of biological and social stages therefore was the need for restraint. The "education" of the faithful would require, he thought, a continuing watchfulness over natural inclinations, for natural impulse always bore the mark of fallenness. For Wesley, the natural was always ambiguous: it reflected the original created harmony but also bore the consequences of the original

133

rebellion against harmony. Such fallenness ensured a dissonance between the natural inclinations and the law of love.

The need for restraint became especially pronounced when Wesley attended to the perplexing demands of human sexuality. Sex was a problem for Wesley, both in his own life and in his movement. For a time he thought that the solution lay in celibacy, but he changed his mind and consequently recommended less demanding forms of restraint. Yet he never felt comfortable with sexuality, and he never overcame his suspicion that it distracted the Christian from higher things.

Few twentieth-century Methodists would share Wesley's understanding of infancy or his methods of rearing children or his attitudes toward marriage. The Methodist tradition has been marked by a transition from Wesley's ideal of restraint to a broader ideal of responsibility. Precisely for that reason, the topics of biological maturation and human sexuality provide a useful illustration of how a tradition can change and yet retain recognizable features.

## THE RESTRAINT OF IMPULSE

For Wesley, the need for restraint began with infancy. He thought that the primary task of Christian parents was to "break the will" of their children and thereby overcome their natural propensities. Wesley believed that every child entered the world bearing the burden of "spiritual disease," which could be overcome only through a "Christian education." Children were naturally prone to atheism, pride, sensuality, dissimulation, and injustice. Only by crushing their "self-will" could parents ensure that their children would not fall prey to their natural disorders: "Break the will of your child, to bring his will into subjection to yours," Wesley urged, "that it may be afterwards subject to the will of God."[4]

Wesley's advice about the rearing of children had little in common with the advice that might appear in a guidebook for twentieth-century parents. He told eighteenth-century mothers and fathers that they should not humor a crying child: "If you give a child what he cries for, you pay him for crying; and then he will certainly cry again." He urged them not to encourage pride in their children: "Almost all parents are guilty of doing this, by praising their children to their face." He recommended that they discourage their children from seeking pleasure in the outward senses, and he criticized indulgent parents who failed to exercise proper restraint:

They cherish "the desire of the flesh," that is, the tendency to seek happiness in pleasing the outward senses, by studying to enlarge the pleasure of tasting in their children to the uttermost: not only giving them before they are weaned other things beside milk, the natural food of children; but giving them both before and after, any sort of meat or drink that they will take. Yea, they entice them, long before nature requires it, to take wine, or strong drink; and provide them with comfits, gingerbread, raisins, and whatever fruit they have a mind to. They feed in them "the desire of the eyes," the propensity to seek happiness in pleasing the imagination, by giving them pretty playthings, glittering toys, shining buckles, or buttons, fine clothes, red shoes, laced hats, needless ornaments, as ribands, necklaces, ruffles; yea, and by proposing any of these as rewards for doing their duty, which is stamping a great value upon them.[5]

In opposition to such indulgence, Wesley said, wise parents would permit their children no food but milk until they are weaned, and even then they would allow only the simplest of foods, mainly vegetables.

Wise parents, moreover, would closely observe servants and grandparents and prevent their exercising any indulgence toward the children. They would give the children no toys or ornaments; allow them no expressions of anger; permit no lying, even in jest, and no cruelty, either to animals or to other children. They would "wean them . . . from all these false ends, habituate them to make God their end in all things; and inure them, in all they do, to aim at knowing, loving, and serving God."[6]

"My own mother had ten children, each of whom had spirit enough," he wrote. "Yet not one of them was ever heard to cry aloud, after it was a year old."[7] Susannah Wesley had indeed begun training her children in a "regular method of living" even during the first months of their lives.

The children were always put into a regular method of living in such things as they were capable of, from their birth; as in dressing and undressing, changing their linen, etc. The first quarter commonly passes in sleep. After that they were, if possible, laid into their cradle awake, and rocked to sleep, and so they were kept rocking till it was time for them to awake. This was done to bring them to a regular course of sleeping, which at first was three hours in the morning and three in the afternoon; afterwards two . . . till they needed none at all. When turned a year old (and some before) they were taught to fear the rod and cry softly, by which means they escaped abundance of correction which they might otherwise have had: and that most odious noise of the crying of children was rarely heard in the house, but the family usually lived in as much quietness as if there had not been a child among them.[8]

Her goal, she said, was to "conquer their will and bring them to an obedient temper."[9]

As the children grew older, she permitted no loud playing, no loud talking, and no conversations with the servants. She saw to it that the children ate three meals a day, but no more. At meals they could not ask aloud for food; they relayed their requests in a whisper to a servant, who then conveyed each request to their mother. Not only did they have to ask parental permission to play with one another, but also they had to take care not to call each other by first names; they could address one another only as "brother" or "sister." Such regulation of childish exuberance would break and restrain the children's wills: "When a child is corrected it must be conquered. . . . And when the will of the child is totally subdued, and it is brought to revere and stand in awe of the parents, then a great many childish follies and inadvertencies may be passed by." By such methods, she hoped to produce children who would commit "no willful transgression."[10] Wesley revered his mother and praised her methods of training her children. He reported that he rendered obedience to her even after he passed his fortieth birthday.[11]

When in 1748 Wesley established the Kingswood School near Bristol, he intended to put such ideas into practice, first by subjecting the students to a rigorous academic regimen and then by ensuring an equally rigorous subjection to the discipline of proper schoolmasters. Through constant oversight of every activity, the masters would form the children into models of holiness. No child was ever to be left alone, beyond the immediate attention of the master. No child was to waste time in play or frivolity. No child was to sleep beyond the hour of four in the morning. The school would be a model of discipline, subordinating the natural impulses always to the higher aims of Christian piety.

Or so Wesley hoped. In fact, his young scholars and their masters constantly disappointed him. His laboratory in the disciplining of the childish soul succeeded only in demonstrating the resistance and resilience of the natural vitalities. Wesley's masters would not crawl out of bed so early every morning and his scholars would not submit to a life without play, even if they had to slip away to the woods to have their way. Wesley grumbled about the resistance: "It must be mended, or ended; for no school is better than the present school." Kingswood later became one of England's national public schools, but it never quite fit the vision of the founder.[12]

Wesley's sense of the need for restraint appeared especially when he touched on the topic of sexual behavior. He recognized the power and complexity of sexual impulse. When he referred to sexuality as a "natural appetite," he meant not to praise its innocence or utility but to indicate its ambiguity. Sexual impulse was a necessary means of fulfilling God's intention for humanity. Yet it was also a troubling distraction, drawing the soul from its proper ends. Wesley respected the Christian traditions of ascetic celibacy, and he never completely abandoned the conviction that voluntary celibacy might well be the highest path for the Christian properly intent on the aims of the larger pilgrimage.

As a child, Wesley assumed that he would never marry because he would never find a woman like his mother. As a young man, he came to believe not only that it was unlawful for an Anglican priest to marry but also that the marriage bed inevitably imposed some degree of "taint" upon the mind. At one point, he resolved upon a lifetime of celibacy, without the distractions or the burdens of marriage.[13]

Wesley told his father in 1735 that one reason for his going to Georgia was his desire to keep away from attractive women. Yet his ambivalence created problems for him even in America. He fell in love with Sophia Hopkey, hinted at marriage, backed away, and then behaved terribly when she married someone else. After his return to England, Wesley gradually changed his mind about celibacy, but it was not until 1748 that he felt fully confident that "a believer might marry, without suffering loss in his soul" and that sexual intercourse in marriage was "undefiled, and no necessary hindrance to the highest perfection." It took a spirited debate at a Methodist conference in London in 1748 to convince him.[14]

Wesley's own marriage in 1751 proved disastrous. Having decided that he "might be more useful in a married state," he joined in matrimony with a merchant's widow named Molly Vazeille. He felt that he truly did love her, and he assured her, in his letters, of his love and affection. His travels, however, placed strain on the marriage. Molly Wesley disliked the long absences; she resented his spiritual direction of pious women, which Wesley conducted in letters of warmth, familiarity, and intimacy; she wearied of his imperious manner. For his part, John Wesley felt aggrieved when his wife secretly opened and read his private letters of spiritual guidance; he was baffled by her intense jealousy; he disapproved of her stern treatment of the servants; he received reports that she spoke ill—even slanderously—of him to others; and he wearied of her own imperious manner. She left him several times, and they were living apart when she died.[15]

The marriage helped to confirm his suspicion that a single life would be preferable for the "happy few" who had the gift for it. He always thought that it would be better "to conquer our natural desires" rather than submit to them, and as late as 1785, he was still worrying that marriage might be a dangerous substitute for the knowledge and love of God. He had no desire to impose celibacy upon his Methodists, but he did feel it important at least to regulate their marriages to the extent of forbidding them to marry unbelievers. In his *Explanatory Notes Upon the New Testament*, he expressed his agreement with Paul that it was "good" not to marry—"so great and many are the advantages of a single life"—even though marriage was often needful "in order to avoid fornication."[16]

He expected his Methodists to exercise restraint both in conceiving their children and in rearing them, and his attitudes toward both sexuality and childhood exemplified his conviction that a disposition of self-denial should guide the Christian through all the passages of life. He emphasized with customary severity the Matthean teaching that lust was tantamount to adultery: "Pull out your eyes," he wrote to the men in his movement, "if you can no otherwise be restrained from lusting after a woman." Expecting his followers to discipline their innermost thoughts, Wesley advised them to avoid delicacy, softness, and excessive sleep, on the grounds that such self-indulgence inflamed the appetites and passions. It is no exaggeration to say that Wesley felt a wariness of sexuality as a threat to the purity of heart that marked the life of love.[17]

He was not entirely lacking, however, in a recognition that sexual union could embody a sense of mutual responsibility and care. He never felt inclined to approve, for example, of celibacy within marriage. "Let not married persons fancy there is any perfection," he wrote, "in living with each other as if they were unmarried."[18]

He eventually recognized, in fact, that marriage, rather than being a barrier on the Christian journey, could deepen the religious life. He came to view the "marriage covenant" as the "closest" of all earthly covenants and instructed married couples that they were to love each other "even as Christ hath loved the church, when he laid down his life for it." Husbands and wives had taken each other "for better or worse," he said, and he urged them to "make the best of each other, seeing as God has joined them together."[19]

Wesley preached on "family religion," observing that the home could become a nursery of faith and love for the spouses, the children, and even the servants. As was typical of the earlier pietist movements which had so deeply touched him during the 1730s, he came to view the family as a resource for mutual encouragement, correction, and instruction, subject always, of course, to the authority of the father as the head of the household.[20]

Wesley thought that he had himself enjoyed a rich family life as one of eleven surviving children, most of whom were sisters. He never speculated, but it is entirely plausible to suggest that his remarkable ability to work closely with women in his later Methodist movement may have been one of the fruits of his own experiences in a largely feminine family dominated by a matriarch. Despite his predilection for strictness in child rearing, Wesley referred to the family as a communion of kindred spirits ideally marked by both faith and love.[21]

In writing about sexuality and the family, therefore, Wesley could move beyond the rigid boundaries of restraint. He could view both as occasions for the exercise of mutual responsibility. It is true that his emphasis on restraint overshadowed his more positive insights; in that regard, his views about the family and sexuality were typical of a viewpoint widely shared in eighteenth-century evangelical circles. Wesley's convictions about breaking the will of children, for example, were no idiosyncrasy but an expression of a consensus among an evangelical subculture in eighteenth-century England and America.[22] Nevertheless, for reasons both temperamental and cultural, Wesley elevated the theme of restraint over the theme of responsibility.

## FROM RESTRAINT TO RESPONSIBILITY

In 1972, the United Methodist Church restated what had become a common Methodist viewpoint: "We recognize that sexuality is a good gift of God, and we believe persons may be fully human only when that gift is acknowledged and affirmed by themselves, the church, and society." On theological grounds, Wesley's tradition had altered his uneven balance of restraint and responsibility. In place of the rhetoric of negative restraint, the Methodists had adopted a notion of "responsible sexuality" that permitted them to interpret human sexual expression as a fulfillment of personality.[23]

For anyone seeking to understand current Methodist views of sexuality, the tradition's movement from restraint to responsibility provides an instructive case study in continuity and change. The 1972 resolution on sexuality came as no sudden revolution. From the beginning of the nineteenth century, Methodists had gradually altered Wesley's views, often justifying the modifications by appealing to characteristic Wesleyan theological motifs. The tradition itself provided the resources to check and correct the views of its founder.

By 1823, Methodist theologians were already beginning to rethink the founder's ideas. Richard Watson spoke of marriage as "the highest, most endearing, and sanctified relation in which two human beings can stand to each other." While he acknowledged that providence called some persons to duties in the church and the world which might better be performed in a single and unfettered life, he argued that the "instincts of nature" revealed marriage to be the general rule for men and women.[24]

Watson showed no reluctance to emphasize the sexual side of marriage. He discovered the foundation of marriage in the divine command to "be fruitful and multiply," and he defined the three ends of marriage as the production of children, the promotion of happiness through affection between children and parents, and the "prevention of fornication." Marriage channeled the power of sexuality, not only by providing a "lawful gratification of the sexual appetite" but also by promoting "mutual affection" between husband and wife.[25]

It became a common Methodist assumption that marriage had its foundation in the "constitutional nature and essential relations of man and woman" and that its primary intention was the "regular and healthy reproduction of the human family." Such a view of marriage presupposed that the chief end of sexual intercourse was the procreation of children. Yet even though the theologians did not say explicitly that sexual union also served the purpose of expressing "reciprocal affection," they did argue that marriage was more than simply an arrangement for reproduction. By grounding marriage on the "instincts and inclinations" and by insisting that it rightly required love and affection between husband and wife, they implied that sexual union might serve to express depths of the relationship other than simply the desire for children. Nevertheless, in the nineteenth century the lingering suspicion of sexuality precluded any development of that implication.[26]

Yet the early nineteenth-century theologians had made the crucial step. Insofar as they argued that one end of marriage was to prevent fornication, they implied, of course, that the institution had the negative function of restraining fallen impulses. They retained something of the older Wesleyan sense of restraint. But by grounding marriage in the instincts and inclinations of human nature, thereby linking it theologically to the doctrine of creation, they also broke away from any lingering special valuation of celibacy. And by beginning to exploit the Pauline idea that husbands and wives stood in a relation like that between Christ and the Church, they suggested a degree of harmony between the common human passages and the larger Christian journey. Because marriage required the husband and wife to attend to mutual "religious edification," the institution became an agency in the journey of salvation.[27]

The accent on responsible sexuality provided a way of re-envisioning the ethical imperatives implicit in human relationships and also a way of recognizing that sexual responsiveness, as one dimension of responsibility, could become an expression of care and not simply a channeling of biological impulse. Meanwhile, the continued accent on restraint maintained the awareness that human sexuality is itself never free from the ambiguity that marks all human activity, and thus cannot be used as a means of escaping that ambiguity.

A brief look at the tradition's changing conceptions of marriage, sexuality, divorce, birth control, and masturbation reveals the direction of Methodist reflection and suggests implications for issues of health and medicine.

### Marriage and Its Sexual Expression

By the late nineteenth century, Methodist theologians were arguing that the purpose of marriage was not only to manifest the continuing creative activity of God but also to embody a covenantal fidelity that symbolized the relation between God and God's faithful people. By the end of the century, Methodists commonly insisted that marriage was a "sacred institution" precisely because it perpetuated both the covenantal and the creative dimensions of God's purposes.

In the judgment of Methodist theologians of the time, however, the procreative function of marriage as a fitting means to produce and nurture children clearly outweighed its covenantal character. After all, they assumed that marriage was an institution through which "one man and one woman will usually have as many children as they can, in a life-time, care for and properly educate." Such an understanding of marriage permitted an affirmation of sexual impulse: "The desire for sex," wrote Miner Raymond in 1879, "is an implanted principle." But the emphasis on the procreative purpose of marriage suggested an exclusively procreative understanding of sexual intercourse.[28]

By the end of the nineteenth century, a few Methodist theologians began to emphasize the covenantal dimension of marriage. Borden Parker Bowne, writing in 1892, acknowledged that "the contents of the notion of marriage spring partly from the physical side of our being and relate to the perpetuation of the race." But he considered this "far from being the whole of the matter, or even its most important factor." Bowne grounded marriage in "the social and affectional nature" of men and women, and he saw its primary aim as the promotion of "moral culture." Marriage was a relationship designed, he thought, to train men and women and their children in the lessons of love, patience, forbearance, and unselfishness.[29]

In the twentieth century, Methodist theologians who wrote about marriage continued to discuss both its covenantal and its procreative aspects, but now the weight increasingly fell on the covenantal. American Methodists spoke of the "sanctity of the marriage covenant which is best expressed by love and mutual support." They expressed the conviction that the blessing of God graced marriage even in the absence of children.[30]

Marriage in this view is a commitment between one man and one woman, designed to nurture and sustain mutual love, responsibility, respect, and fidelity. The birth and nurture of children remain a central purpose of marriage but not its only purpose. In effect, the Methodist churches have ceased to identify the creative side of marriage solely with procreative sexual union. And they have recognized the ways in which sexual expression can confirm and deepen the covenantal relationship. An English theologian can write that "the relational and procreative functions of sex are equally rooted in the creative purpose of God, and neither is subordinated to the other," adding that "the instincts and impulses of sex are part of the divine order of nature." An American United Methodist Conference can insist that "we view our sexuality in the light of the goodness of this creation, believing it to be intended for the fulfillment of personality as well as for procreation."[31]

In connecting sexual expression and the covenantal side of marriage, the later Methodists have affirmed two traditional Wesleyan convictions. First, they have agreed that sexual intercourse should occur within the marriage bond. Such an agreement reflects both a Methodist understanding of biblical tradition and an awareness that sexual intercourse, as a profound and compelling human experience, can easily become an instrument of exploitation if not informed by an intention of lasting care and commitment. Methodist conferences have recognized that sexual relationships within marriage can also be exploitative, but they have remained especially sensitive to the possibilities of pain and exploitation in sexual intercourse that occurs without the concrete commitments symbolized and undertaken through marriage.

Second, later Methodists have agreed that the covenantal breadth of marriage extends beyond the narrow limits of two personalities. A Methodist General Conference in 1968 insisted that "the sex act is never isolated within the separate personalities of participants or within their total relationship as persons." Just as Methodists believe that marriage is not simply an end in itself but also a means directed toward larger purposes, so also they believe that the decision to join with another person in sexual intercourse can never be isolated from the larger pattern of decisions, commitments, and relationships that define both the Christian community and the wider human community.[32]

Early Methodists expressed that awareness by forbidding church members to marry persons who did not share in the Christian faith. The churches have abandoned that rule, but they have kept the conviction that both marriage and sexual union occur within larger communities—of parents, families, friends, other Christians, other persons—that rightfully advance a claim for respect and care, and within larger commitments that orient our lives. To conceive of sexual expression merely as a means of self-fulfillment is to ignore those communities and commitments and thus to turn sexuality into an instrument of isolation.[33]

In linking marriage and the family to such values as mutual support and nurture, the later Methodist tradition has reflected the social and economic change from the family-craft economy of the eighteenth century to the impersonal bureaucratic economies of the twentieth. That economic transition created firm boundaries between the domestic and the economic, as the household became not the locus of production but a retreat from the rigors of the marketplace. It also established sharper divisions between men and women, as the new organization of trades, crafts, and factories in the nineteenth century left urban women at home in domestic rather than public productive roles. Furthermore, it intensified the expectation that the primary purpose of marriage and sexuality was to fulfill human needs for security, intimacy, and mutuality.

The result was increasing dissatisfaction when the family could not bear the full weight of the new burden it was expected to carry. The ensuing stresses have created new conceptions of therapeutic care among Methodist pastoral theologians, who now often insist that pastoral counselors should conceive of their task as a ministry not simply to individual persons but also to their families, and who sometimes advise that family members be included in pastoral counseling sessions.

### Divorce

John Wesley permitted divorce only for adultery or the danger of a loss of life. Such a position remained typical of Methodism throughout the nineteenth century. Borden Parker Bowne was still insisting in 1892 that divorce should be granted only for adultery, gross fraud, or groundless and long-continuing desertion, and he believed that the right to remarry should be accorded only to the innocent partner, lest the church "encourage crime."[34]

In 1904 a Methodist General Conference elaborated a position that would define the church's stance for half a century:

> No divorce, except for adultery, shall be regarded by the Church as lawful; and no minister shall solemnize marriage in any case where there is a

divorced wife or husband living; but this rule shall not be applied to the innocent party to a divorce for the cause of adultery, nor to divorced parties seeking to be reunited in marriage.[35]

After the end of World War II, however, Methodists gradually altered their positions.

In 1946, English Methodists ruled that divorce was possible for church members if the marriage were broken beyond the possibility of restoration, and in 1961 they gave their pastors the latitude to decide whether it was appropriate to solemnize the marriage of a person who had suffered divorce. They argued that "a complete ban on remarriage tilts the scales too far towards legalism in morals and religion; [but that] remarriage in all cases sways the balance too far towards successive polygamy."[36]

Other Methodists had begun by 1961 to move away from a sharp dichotomy between the innocent and the guilty, to view divorce as symptomatic of deeper difficulties, and to recognize the right of divorced persons to remarry. The General Conference of the United Methodist Church permitted ministers to perform such ceremonies when, after counseling, they believed that the divorced person was aware of the reasons the previous marriage failed, was preparing to make the proposed marriage truly Christian, and was willing to allow sufficient time for adequate counseling and preparation.[37]

*Contraception*

The most dramatic reflection of changing Methodist attitudes toward marriage and sexuality came as the tradition altered its stance toward contraception. During the early decades of the twentieth century, Methodists remained silent or antagonistic toward the proponents of birth control. By the 1930s, though, the church's theologians and conferences began to support planned parenthood, and in 1939 the English Methodist "Declaration on the Christian View of Marriage and the Family" announced the church's tentative approval.

The announcement did not come without a struggle. The conference heard objections from delegates who argued that the sole purpose of marriage was "that the work of creation might go on," and from other delegates who contended that such matters as contraception "ought not to be talked about" by religious groups. The opponents argued that the Declaration had abandoned a traditional Wesleyan understanding of marriage as being intended for "the procreation of children in harmony with the will of God" and had adopted a view of sexual intercourse as being intended "for personal pleasure without reference to God."[38]

The caution of the Declaration revealed the intensity of feeling about the issue, and the statement acknowledged the conflicting viewpoints. It noted that many Christians thought that the use of artificial means to prevent conception contravened both the natural order and the spirit of the Christian religion. But it also recognized that others thought contraception was a gift of God, through science, that would permit both the enhancing of marriage as a spiritual and physical union of two persons and the enhancing of parenthood as a responsible task realistically undertaken.

The Declaration concluded that no explicit command of Scripture could be cited for or against either position, and it refused to pass an "unqualified judgment" on either of the two contrasting views. On the one hand, it noted that contraceptive methods made it possible to relieve the strain of inhibition and to avoid the suffering of too-frequent pregnancy. On the other, it cautioned against the possibility that the easy availability of contraceptive devices might develop a "sensual habit of mind" and impair self-control. It concluded that "conception-control commends itself more to the Christian judgment when it is associated, not with the negative purpose of the refusal of parenthood or the undue limitation of families, but with the positive aim of producing the healthiest family in the healthiest possible way."[39]

The proponents of birth control believed not only that the "careful and improvident begetting of children" was wrongful to the children and to the social order but also that "abstinence from sexual intercourse [could] frustrate the relational ends of marriage," and that for both reasons contraceptive devices were beneficial. But they were not abandoning the older Wesleyan view that marriage had procreative ends. They were arguing simply that birth control could enhance even the procreative side of marriage by ensuring that parents could make responsible decisions about procreation. Thus they were suggesting that responsible procreation might require more than simply a reliance on biological rhythms in the organism.[40]

In 1956, the largest of the American Methodist churches announced its conviction that planned parenthood, practiced in Christian conscience, fulfilled rather than violated the will of God. The announcement reflected the dawning awareness that population growth threatened human lives and values, and also the traditional Methodist insistence that God's saving presence in the world both elicited and empowered responsible decision.

In the 1750s, in the controversies over grace and freedom, the Methodists had insisted on the integrity of the human response to God's gracious invitation. In the 1950s, in the controversy over birth control, the Methodists argued that God's larger purposes in the world also required and empowered responsible decision.

> We take this stand [for planned parenthood] in the conviction that God requires human, responsible choice in every matter of moral decision, including such grave matters as the issues of birth and death. We believe it is the will of God that every child born into the world should be wanted, loved, cared for, and reared with opportunities for physical and spiritual health and growth toward mature personality. Apart from responsible parenthood this is impossible. We believe, furthermore, that planned parenthood has an affirmative as well as a negative aspect, and that married couples able to accept the responsibilities of parenthood should not avoid them for selfish reasons.[41]

In 1961 the English Methodists revised their earlier statement, abandoning its equivocation and forthrightly approving the use of contraceptive devices as long as they were "acceptable to both husband and wife."[42]

Such statements represented the emerging consensus in the tradition that the relational and procreative functions of sex were equally rooted in the creative purposes of God, and that God's creative presence could not be bound within the sphere of biology. Insofar as sexual union contributed to the intimacy and depth of the relationship between a husband and a wife, the union embodied the creative presence of God. And what had in 1939 been an equivocal permission became by 1976 a positive duty: "Each couple," declared the United Methodist Church, "has the right and the duty prayerfully and responsibly to control conception according to their circumstances."[43]

The stronger statement in 1976 represented, in part, the fruits of the earlier Methodist position that marriage and sexual union were not accommodations to fallenness but embodiments of God's creative presence. Later Methodist theologians combined that positive evaluation of sexuality with the claim that divine creativity permeated various spheres of life, not simply the limited sphere of biological propagation. The result was the recognition that the relational and the procreative levels of sexual union overlapped, not only in the sense that responsible procreation implied relational commitment, but also in the sense that the engendering of relational intimacy could also be an expression of the creative presence of God.

As early as 1943 the theologian Albert Knudson was arguing that sexual union did not exist simply for procreation: "If it did," he said, "one would hardly expect that the need of sex expression would be as relatively permanent as it is. The nonperiodic character of passion suggests that sexual intercourse not only does have the purpose of procreation but was itself designed by the Creator to be a means by which married couples express their love for one another."[44]

Even that judgment assumes that the exhibition of God's presence and will in the fixed and relatively predictable stabilities of the biological order is a more reliable clue to appropriate behavior than is the manifestation of God's presence and will in the changing historical order—which might require greater sensitivity to such contingencies as the press of population growth on the resources that sustain a livable existence. It assumes that nature's way—and nature's way alone—is God's way.

Such an assumption, carried to its logical conclusion, would preclude any therapeutic intervention designed to impede a natural process. The Methodist tradition has therefore supplemented that naturalistic argument for contraception with the further contention that faithfulness to God's larger purpose requires the exercise of human responsibility. To the extent that contraceptive methods are responsible means of strengthening a marriage in which two people care for each other and for a wider community, the use of such methods can be viewed as a requirement implicit in the command to love one another.

Methodists have concluded, then, that sexual union can express the creative intention of God even in absence of any intent that it produce children. They have also concluded that responsible care for the neighbor, and for the unborn child, might require forthrightly facing the reality that sexual union often occurs outside the boundaries of marriage, among persons who lack either the capacity for relational commitment or the ability to care for children. In facing that reality, some of them have agreed that the use of contraceptive devices can at least reduce the chances of suffering among unwanted children.

An American General Conference in 1976 therefore concluded that every person, regardless of age, should have a right to contraceptive information. The right, however, is clearly subordinate to the responsibility. It would be more in keeping with the tradition to insist that every person has the responsibility to refrain from harming another person; that careless sexual union brings a significant risk of harm not only for the partners in the union but also for the possible unwanted child; and that the use of contraceptive devices can at least diminish the risk of bringing a third person into the realm of harm. The right to contraceptive information is compelling insofar as it makes possible even a minimal reduction in the possibility of harm to a child.[45]

### Masturbation

Finally, the transition in Methodist attitudes toward masturbation serves as another instance of the movement from negative restraint to a broader conception of responsibility. Wesley shared the popular eighteenth-century medical and religious conception of masturbation as a dangerous form of self-abuse. He not only wrote a treatise—*A Word to Whom It May Concern*—against the practice, but he also mistakenly understood masturbation as "the sin of Onan" and frequently warned against any habit, such as excessive sleep or delicacy, that might encourage the sin. Unaware that Onan's transgression recorded in Genesis 38:9 was very probably the interruption of coitus motivated by Onan's unwillingness to "give offspring to his brother," Wesley believed that the Scripture provided a direct injunction against masturbation.[46]

Methodist theologians in the nineteenth century spoke of masturbation as a "solitary vice" that was detrimental to health, destructive of intellect, and ruinous to morals. Their jeremiads against the practice reflected both a quasi-ascetic attitude toward sexual impulse and an acceptance of popular medical conceptions entertained by reputable physicians. In any case, negative judgments on the practice persisted well into the twentieth century.[47]

In 1931, however, Leslie Weatherhead published the popular guidebook *The Mastery of Sex Through Psychology and Religion*, which discussed courtship, marriage, intercourse, birth control, and various other topics, including masturbation. Weatherhead retained many earlier attitudes toward the practice; he felt, for instance, that lustful thoughts during masturbation rendered it sinful. But he also concluded that "the act in itself is neither moral nor immoral. It is the non-biological use of a part of the body for the purpose of obtaining enjoyment."[48]

According to Weatherhead, the physical effects of masturbation were negligible. Its psychological effects could be damaging insofar as it produced undue guilt, but this was because of "the false emotions with which it has been surrounded; emotions, it must be added, the intensity of which are out of all proportions to the seriousness of the habit." The book elicited considerable praise and substantial animosity, but it represented the current state of medical opinion in 1931—Weatherhead observed that he had consulted as many as six eminent medical authorities on the topic of masturbation—and it signaled the emergence of a new attitude within the tradition.[49]

In dealing with such a topic as masturbation, in short, the Methodists have remained open to the wisdom of physicians and psychologists. A brief survey of the textbooks used in courses on sexuality for Methodist young people in the later twentieth century reveals an attitude quite unlike Wesley's. The writers recognize that over 90 percent of males and 50 to 60 percent of females engage in masturbation at one time or another in their lives. They assert that masturbation harms neither the body nor the mind and that it sometimes helps young people relieve sexual tensions that they cannot relieve in any other way. "There are no grounds for guilt feelings," advises one text. "One need have no worry about excessiveness, since the body will take care of this by simply not responding."[50]

The texts labor to dispel misconceptions and hence they avoid subtleties. A more subtle analysis would probably suggest that masturbation, like any other sexual activity, reflects always the ambiguity that attends our humanity. Its meaning cannot be reduced to its biological function. The feelings that accompany masturbation always reflect broader attitudes toward the self, toward sexuality, and toward other persons. It can represent a retreat into solitude, or it can become a realistic means of handling sexual impulse.

In keeping with the medical opinion of our own era, Methodist writers tend not to worry much about masturbation; they are more likely to view it as a normal and acceptable human activity. But they are not likely to view it simply as an isolated physical act: like any other human activity, it accumulates meanings that extend well beyond physical boundaries. Pastors and theologians are far more likely to be concerned about those meanings, which vary from person to person, than they are about older taboos.

In their conceptions of marriage and sexuality, divorce, contraception, and masturbation, then, Methodist theologians have exhibited a transition from restraint to responsibility. Their judgments about specific activities have changed dramatically throughout the past two centuries, but the changes have reflected some continuing affirmations.

Methodists have found it useful to retain the traditional Wesleyan affirmation that the creation, including the created body with its strange and fascinating organs and impulses, is good. They have found new uses for the traditional insistence that human decision and responsibility have a prominent place in God's larger purposes. They have returned often to the Wesleyan doctrine of the image of God, with its suggestion that a person is a unique creation, deserving of respect and care. They have retained the Wesleyan view of love as a gracious gift which draws us beyond ourselves and throws all human activity into new perspective. They have not abandoned the larger conception of the Christian life as a journey which invests marriage and sexuality with purposes beyond themselves.

Finally, they have also not abandoned the grain of wisdom to be found even in the exaggerated sense of restraint that makes Wesley's struggles over marriage and sexuality seem so distant from us. It was only a grain of wisdom; few Methodists today would look to John Wesley for a rounded and complete conception of marriage. But hidden somewhere within Wesley's tortured admonitions of restraint was an awareness of the ambiguity that marks every human activity. In place of a romantic naturalism which celebrates vitality and physical exuberance as unambiguously good and joyous, the religious traditions still are willing to insist that the recognition of ambiguity can provide both a richer and a more humane vision of human sexuality, not because they continue to insinuate that sex is bad, but rather because they can see that sex is complicated.

## RESTRAINT AND RESPONSIBILITY REVISITED

Wesley's view of human sexuality was more than merely a symptom of repressive asceticism. Wesley believed that restraint, narrowly conceived, was necessary inasmuch as sexual inclination distracted attention from the commitments necessary to sustain the work of the Church.

The movement in the nineteenth and twentieth centuries toward a broader conception of sexuality did not entail any wholesale abandonment of restraint but rather its reinterpretation, accomplished by subsuming it within the larger ideal of responsibility and responsiveness. It is fair to say that most Wesleyan theologians find sexuality ambiguous in the way that any deep and good human reality is ambiguous: because of its depth and goodness, it bears greater potential for both benefit and harm than do shallower and lesser realities.

Theodore Jennings, a systematic theologian in the Seminario Metodista de Méjico in Mexico City, expresses that sense of ambiguity when he observes that "the more overtly sexual our relationships become, the more perilous they become as well":

> Whatever proclivities toward a Manichean libel of God's creation and its goodness we may discover in the "puritanical" streams of Judeo-Christian traditions, and however much we may deplore and seek to correct these proclivities, we must also see that here at least the seriousness of sexuality was recognized. However much we may wish to assert the goodness and even the playfulness of sexuality (I remain persuaded that we both may and must assert this against all defamations of God's gifts), we must not forget that we assert this in the face of a fallen condition in which sexuality has become perilous, fraught with the temptation to do violence to one another.[51]

For Jennings, then, sexual relationships are ambiguous, if for no other reason than that they place us in close physical and psychic proximity to one another. Consequently, they both offer us a distinctive occasion for joyful and playful mutuality and tempt us to reduce each other to an instrument for the realization of narcissistic desire.

## Abortion

In our own era, the awareness of that ambiguity has been most acute in the debates over abortion. Those debates have covered the whole range of ethical and theological issues that emerged in the earlier discussions of sexuality and the family. In that sense, the debates over abortion have continued earlier lines of reflection about sexuality, the family, and contraception. But the abortion controversy also took the Methodist tradition by surprise.

Until recently, the familiar texts in ethics and theology largely ignored the issue, and Albert Outler observed in 1973 that even ten years earlier the results of any discussion would have been foreclosed by the prevailing sentiment within the denomination. Within a few years after Outler's observation, however, the Women's Division of the Board of Global Ministries of the United Methodist Church entered as one of the plaintiffs in a federal court case opposing a governmental decision to cut off expenditures for abortions by women on welfare programs. Their participation in the case resulted partly from a feeling that the governmental decision was unfair and inequitable, but it also reflected the division of opinion within the tradition about the purpose and morality of abortion.

The weight of opinion in the Methodist tradition falls heavily against any claim that abortion is simply a medical procedure or a means of birth control comparable to other contraceptive methods or a "right" that overwhelms deeper moral considerations. Methodists in England, for instance, have agreed that "abortion as a means of family limitation is condemned on the ground that when successful, it involves the destruction of human life, and when unsuccessful, the risk of a grave injury in body and mind to mother and child."[52] Yet the weight of opinion also refuses to impose an absolute moral restriction against abortion, as if the value of the life of the unborn child prevailed against every other consideration. The issue of abortion bears the mark of the ambiguity that characterizes any serious human decision, but because abortion always takes away life, the Methodist tradition has been willing to accept it only as a tragic possibility when life is already in conflict with life.

Some Methodist theologians distinguish sharply between life as biological sustenance and life as a qualitative richness of potential experience, and the sharper the distinction, the more likely is the theologian to justify aborting a fetus which is destined for a life seemingly devoid of the capacity to receive love and care. But the Methodist churches have made it clear that they do not consider the fetus to be simply a collection of living tissue, analogous to any other appendage of the woman's body. Both theologians and church resolutions have insisted that the fetus must be considered at least as a potential person and that even the potentiality for personhood distinguishes it as a creature worthy of care and respect.

A brief survey of arguments among Methodist theologians reveals a consistent appropriation of three doctrinal themes from the Wesleyan heritage: the image of God, grace, and responsibility. Of course, the theologians do not return to such themes only because they happen to have occupied a prominent place in early Wesleyan theology; each has a time-honored history in the broader Christian and Jewish traditions. But for whatever reason, all three doctrines—of creation in the image of God, of the gracious character of human reality, and of the human capacity for responsible decision—have had a place in Methodist arguments about abortion.

The doctrine of creation in the image of God stands behind debates about the sanctity of personhood and the identity of the fetus as a person. Methodist theologians have reached no consensus about the vexing question of when the fetus can rightly be called a "person." Some attempt to specify a temporal moment within the process of gestation. Paul Ramsey, for example, has urged theologians to define personhood biologically as a specifiable development in the morphology of the embryonic fetus. Although he recognizes that any such definition requires informed judgment, about which conscientious persons can disagree, he has suggested that a good case can be made for locating the origin of the specifically human either at the moment when conception produces a distinct genotype or at the point of segmentation, when the functional organ systems come into being. His chief concern is that theologians not define personhood with psychological and social criteria that place both the fetus and the unwanted newborn in peril.[53]

Other Methodist theologians contend that every decision about the biological origin of personhood is arbitrary. But most have agreed that the doctrine of creation in the image of God affirms that the fetus embodies a divine intention, that it is on the way to full personhood, and that it must therefore be accorded the respect and care we would offer to any other person. Such an argument is plausible for Methodists because their tradition has insisted that every person, of whatever age or condition, embodies a divine intention and that almost all of us are merely traveling toward full personhood. To discount a life because it has not reached the fullness of which it is capable is to discount almost every life.[54]

The tradition, nevertheless, recognizes that creation in the image of God also renders sacred the life and health of the pregnant woman and that the protection of that sacredness might require the killing of the fetal life. The fetus bears no absolute right over against the pregnant woman, and if the fetal life becomes, tragically, a form of aggression against the life or health of the mother, then the tragic choice to kill the fetus might become the responsible decision. Some Methodist theologians have also contended that when pregnancy results from rape or incest, the need to protect the victimized woman might outweigh the imperative to protect the fetus.[55]

Such a choice is viewed as tragic because of the presupposition in the tradition that every life is a gift. Outler has argued that for a Christian "the primal origins, the continuing ground and final ends of human life are truly transcendental."[56] If each life is a gift, not an achievement, then each life is of comparable worth. No utilitarian calculation of social usefulness can suffice for a judgment about the ultimate disposal of a human life.

Even so, on certain occasions the capacity to accept the gracious and giftlike character of life is overwhelmed by circumstance. When severe defects in the fetal organism allow it no hope of ever exhibiting signs of distinctively human life, and thus no hope of meaningfully receiving the love and care that represent and embody God's grace, some Methodist theologians argue that abortion might be justifiable.

Harmon Smith of Duke University has contended, for example, that mercy and reason can foreclose the birth of nascent life which is or promises to be severely deformed, defective, or disadvantaged.[57] Probably many Methodist theologians would share that judgment, with the proviso that in such a case, the primary consideration should be the proper exercise of responsibility on behalf of the fetus, rather than the convenience of the parents.

On the whole, Methodist theologians have tended to talk more about concrete responsibility than about abstract rights. The primary question is not so much "How do I assert my rights?" as it is "How do I exercise my responsibility?" Because the Christian tradition has called especially for the exercise of care and responsibility for the weak, Methodist theologians have been sensitive to the plight of the helpless. And that has created a wariness about any facile resort to abortion. "Care for the unborn," writes Outler, "is a mutuality between the weaker and stronger. It is the essence of every relationship of unselfish love."[58]

To be sure, Christian moral decision entails also the obligation to inquire about appropriate responsibility to and for the pregnant woman, the father, the wider family, persons seeking to adopt a child, the Christian community, and the wider human community. The Christian ethic also requires each of those persons or groups to ask about its responsibility to and for the others. But the claim that we are responsible persons—a claim dear to Wesley's heart—raises the pertinent question of the nature of our responsibility for the helpless.

In the United States, many Methodists have supported the carefully defined legal right to abortion, though without assuming that legal rights and moral warrants are necessarily the same. A statement adopted by a United Methodist General Conference in 1972 reflects much of the substance and tone of current Methodist thought:

> Our belief in the sanctity of unborn life makes us reluctant to approve abortion. But we are equally bound to respect the sacredness of the life and well-being of the mother, for whom devastating damage may result from an unacceptable pregnancy. In continuity with past Christian teachings, we recognize tragic conflicts of life with life that may justify abortion. We call our fellow Christians to a searching and prayerful inquiry into the sorts of conditions that for us warrant abortion.[59]

Most Methodists have refused to declare either that "all abortions are murders" or that they are "medical procedures without moral significance." To many it seems that they are, rather, ambiguous human dilemmas requiring the thoughtful and sensitive exercise of moral responsibility.[60]

### Homosexuality

Methodist theologians have also recognized the ambiguities presented by the current debates over homosexuality. John Wesley saw homosexual behavior as simply a sign of original sin, and he believed that the Roman tolerance of homosexuality was a signal mark of the sinfulness of the ancient world. But after a governmental study in 1957 in England led to the abolition of laws in that country against homosexual relations between consenting adults, and after the emergence in the late 1960s of a vigorous gay-rights movement within American religious communities, the Methodist tradition, like others, had to reexamine the issue. By 1972, the churches faced divisive debate.

The debate in the United Methodist Church resulted in a statement that homosexual practice was "incompatible with Christian teaching." But that statement did not stand alone, and the debate also produced an interesting combination of theological and medical arguments. On one level, Methodists looked at the question of homosexuality as a therapeutic matter. In 1968, an American general conference referring to "persons who are troubled and broken by sexual problems" included homosexuality among the problems. The conference urged that such persons be brought under the care of health and human development services rather than being subjected to penal and correctional institutions.[61]

Four years later, the medical diagnoses faded into the background, and the conference spoke merely of the need to accord homosexuals "spiritual and emotional care." The change reflected, in part, the indecision among psychiatrists and psychologists about whether homosexuality was to be viewed as a personality disorder. But it also reflected a theological judgment. In trying to discern an appropriate course, Methodists turned to the biblical traditions, and the broader implications of biblical teachings led them back to familiar theological guidelines.[62]

The United Methodist Church concluded that "homosexuals no less than heterosexuals are persons of sacred worth, who need the ministry and guidance of the church in their struggles for human fulfillment, as well as the spiritual and emotional care of a fellowship which enables reconciling relationships with God, with others and with self."[63] But while calling for church and society to protect the human and civil rights of homosexuals, Methodists have also refused to condone homosexual practice. Four successive General Conferences of the denomination have passed the same statement on homosexuality, with its distinction between the homosexual's rights as person and citizen, and homosexual "practice" as "incompatible" with Christian sexual morality.

Such a position offered an alternative to the earlier dubious efforts at medical diagnosis in church resolutions, which seemed increasingly problematic in view of the current confusion of medical judgments among psychiatrists and psychologists. The position also allows the church to acknowledge the ambiguity in the issue of homosexuality. Some Methodists argue that a homosexual relationship can serve as an expression of mutual care; others argue, however, that the widespread practice of homosexuality seems not to encourage the stability and commitment that the church has sought to promote as the deeper meaning of sexual union. Still others have insisted that homosexual practice appears to be especially susceptible to a pattern of casual encounters and exploitation.

The debate, in short, has not in recent years rested on efforts at medical diagnosis but on broader ethical considerations. As a result of that debate, the church has refused to encourage homosexual practice. But it has insisted that such a refusal need not become a condemnation of persons who find in themselves a predominant inclination toward homosexuality. Such, at least, is the tenuous balance that has emerged in the pronouncements of one Methodist denomination.

## Adolescence and Aging

The transitions in attitudes toward sexuality have corresponded to a broader change in Methodist conceptions of the natural passages. By the late nineteenth century, pious Methodists were no longer set on breaking the wills of their sinful offspring. They were beginning to think of childhood and adolescence as periods of maturation during which the religious feelings came to fruition along with other capacities. Such groups as the Epworth League symbolized the new insight that young people shared distinctive outlooks and emotions and that the church could best guide them by accepting and encouraging their youthful exuberance.

The Epworth League, founded in 1889 for Methodist youth, originated in the awareness that adolescence brought sexual and social changes which created emotional and intellectual ferment. The organization's primary purpose was to cultivate the spiritual life of young Christians, but its founders also argued that it promoted mental health by guiding young boys and girls through the stages of socialization, from solitude to membership in gangs and cliques and then toward larger communities.

Some of its later proponents explicitly defended the Epworth League as an agency that guided youth from negative restraint toward a larger sense of responsibility:

> Restraint has its value in moral education, but its place is earlier and its worth inferior. "Thou shalt not" belongs to a stage of religious development much earlier than that of "Ye shall be holy, for I am holy." Even this is far below "Ye are my friends. All things that I have heard from my Father I have made known unto you." The social impulse of sex craves responsibility because it is one of the conditions of home making and the care of offspring. In religion the same impulse takes the form of volunteer activities.... Leadership is developed through the bearing of responsibility and through self-direction. The Epworth League is organized upon this principle.[64]

The Epworth League eventually gave way to a variety of later organizations for Methodist youth, but all of them retained the conviction that adolescence constituted a distinguishable stage of life, which brought special problems of mental and spiritual health. When Methodist pastoral theologians offered advice about child rearing in the twentieth century, therefore, they were far more likely to warn against narrow severity than to encourage it. They emphasized instead the need to be attentive to the organic changes that marked the stages of childhood development.[65]

By the twentieth century, moreover, Methodists were finding that their ethical insistence on the "worth and dignity of all persons" required that they attend not simply to the vitalities of the young but also to the needs and the wisdom of the old.[66] The transition in attitudes toward aging and the aged can be charted by noting once again the increasing emphasis on the theme of responsibility.

Wesley could serve as an example not only because he remained active throughout almost all his eighty-seven years, and not only because he worked to provide homes for "feeble, aged widows," but also because he recognized the special usefulness of the aged as visitors of the sick and leaders in the societies. He thought that older people could be beneficial visitors because in eighteenth-century English society they retained, so he believed, a distinctive "authority."[67]

Throughout the early nineteenth century, the leaders of Methodism ascribed a special sanctity and authority to the elderly saints in the faith. Typical of their rhetoric, however, was an idealized portrait of old age which recognized its "many miseries" while concentrating on the opportunities of the elderly to improve their "contemplative habits" and review their lives in preparation for their death: "The aged Christian is truly tranquil." Explicit in this idealizing piety, moreover, was often the recommendation that older persons should "retreat from care" and "leave the cares which would encumber." To the degree that this theme of retreat found expression, the tradition lost sight of Wesley's sense that the aged might need to accept some continuing responsibility, such as visiting the sick, even at the risk of having to bear with encumbrances.[68]

Methodists did not lose sight of Wesley's example in providing homes for older persons who could no longer manage alone. As early as 1845, Stephen Smith, a local preacher and philanthropist in the African Methodist Episcopal Church, founded a Home for Aged and Infirm Colored People at Philadelphia, and by 1850 other Methodist groups began to build homes for the aged, mainly from a sense that they should care for their own people. The Methodist Home for the Aged and Infirm, erected in Philadelphia in 1865, was intended for "worthy aged and infirm members of the Methodist Episcopal Church." Only later did Methodists view their homes for the aged as expressions of a sense of responsibility for the larger community.[69]

The theme of responsibility emerged again in the late nineteenth century, with a different twist. The Methodist advocates of the social gospel insisted in their Social Creed of 1908 that the larger society bore a responsibility to its older members. Their statement on the "Social Ideals of the Churches" urged that private and public agencies join to ensure "suitable provision for the old age of the workers." The proponents of the social gospel in American Methodism therefore gave enthusiastic support, almost three decades later, to the passage of the Social Security Act of 1935.[70]

In the 1940s the Methodist Church assigned a full-time worker to the study of programs for older persons, and between 1946 and 1948, the church joined with the Federal Council of Churches in its first full-scale study of the ministry of the church to older people. Led by Paul B. Maves and J. Lennart Cedarleaf, the researchers conducted programs and studies in thirteen Methodist churches. One result was the publication by Maves and Cedarleaf in 1949 of *Older People and the Church*, which went beyond conclusions about spiritual growth to include questions about mental health, biological and cognitive changes in older people, health care, and personality characteristics of the elderly.[71]

They urged that churches and social agencies become more responsible for the needs of the elderly. Pointing out the problems of securing inexpensive health care, for instance, they argued that "more clinics, which are cheaper, tend to mean fewer hospital-bed-days, which are more expensive." They also insisted that effective clinics would place their emphasis on preventive services. Noting the problems of housing, they argued that both public and private agencies needed to invest more in institutions, and they praised the Board of Hospitals and Homes of the Methodist Church for helping to ensure that as early as 1948 the denomination had already constructed 55 homes for older people, a number which would, by the 1980s, increase to 234.[72]

One of the useful conclusions in the study by Maves and Cedarleaf was that older people usually sought not a retreat from the world but an opportunity to work and serve. "It is fallacious," they wrote, "to assume that older people want to be relieved of responsibility and made comfortable in order that they be free completely of strain of any kind." They gave careful attention, therefore, to the ways in which small groups in churches could help older people continue to assume responsibility for themselves and for other persons. They thought that the churches could help the elderly rethink goals and values, find resources, and learn to handle conflict and stress.[73]

Those who wanted to help the elderly continue to assume such responsibility, they said, had to recognize that increasing years did bring changes in personality and behavior. Older people moved at a slower tempo; they often sharpened their own sense of individuality, which led others sometimes to consider them eccentric; they could be excessively responsive in expressing love or gratitude, a trait which often hid a diminished sense of worth; and they needed to find persons willing to listen to them as they tried to reshape their lives in the light of old memories and new tasks. But none of these traits meant that the elderly should, as a group, be urged to withdraw or retreat from assuming appropriate responsibilities.[74] Just as the recent tradition has accented responsibility in its views of sexuality and youth, so also its modern formative study of aging returned to the same theme.

The Methodist tradition, for obvious reasons, has been especially open to developmental depictions of human existence. Developmental psychologies have seemed to bear a faint analog to the traditional Wesleyan conception of religious growth. And insofar as those psychologies have affirmed the movement from narrow restraint toward subtle judgment and the capacity for responsible decision, the Methodist tradition has seen them as secular allies in the effort to understand the religious journey.

The tradition, therefore, has struggled with the themes of restraint and responsibility, and that struggle continues. Wesley would not approve of all the conclusions, but he would surely recognize the persistence of appeal to the doctrinal themes of creation, grace, and responsibility. And he would probably have to admit that some of the changes have resulted not from an abandonment of those themes but from continued reflection on them.

# ·7·

# Caring and Well-Being

Wesley created his Methodist societies for men and women who had "a desire to flee from the wrath to come, to be saved from their sins." When he made the rules for those societies, he indicated that they had a dual intent: members were to evidence their desire of salvation "first, by doing no harm, by avoiding evil in every kind.... [and] secondly, by doing good, by being in every kind merciful after their power."[1]

Wesley also assigned a dual purpose to the small classes in which members of the societies were to meet at least once each week: they were for both reproof and comfort, he said, "as occasion may require." And when he created the smaller "bands," he spoke of them also as having a twofold purpose: we meet in bands, he said, "to confess our faults to one another and pray one for another that we may be healed."[2]

The institutional structures of early Methodism thus maintained a pattern of alternation between discipline and support, restraint and responsibility, reproof and comfort, confession of fault and prayer for healing. They maintained a dialectic of limit and possibility.

The Methodist conception of caring has often, though not always, preserved that dialectic. The early Wesleyan optimism about the possibility of entire sanctification had its counterpart in the early Wesleyan realism about the need for Christians to recognize the limits imposed by finitude and sinfulness. All Methodists were expected to attend the band sessions and evidence a willingness to "be told of all [their] faults."[3]

In the early tradition, the understanding of the dialectic came almost exclusively from scriptural and theological sources. When eighteenth-century Methodists thought about the relation between caring and curing, moreover, they usually had in mind only the expectation that members of classes should visit the sick. But gradually Methodists began to explore other conceptual sources for understanding care and other practical forms of caring and curing.

By the twentieth century, medical practice exerted a strong influence on theological conceptions of caring within Methodism. The pastoral theologian Carroll Wise, writing in 1966, spoke for many Methodist clergy and laity when he testified to the contribution the medical profession had made to the religious community: "I, for one," he said, "make no apologies to anyone for turning to the medical profession to learn something about the healing process."[4] In the preceding chapters of this book, religious and theological understandings of medicine and health have been the focus. In this concluding chapter, the emphasis falls on how the tradition has drawn on medical theory and practice to modify and expand its conceptions of caring. The development of new therapeutic skills and theories in the twentieth century has altered the terms of the debate among Methodist theologians about the proper balance of possibility and limit in Christian care.

## LIMIT AND POSSIBILITY

John Wesley's chief contribution to Christian care was his innovative use of small groups for spiritual formation. After establishing his first United Society in London in 1739, Wesley divided each society into classes of about twelve persons, led by a layperson who was to assist them in fulfilling their intention to do good, refrain from harm, and evidence their desire for salvation. He then organized smaller bands, in which members were encouraged to assist and confide in one another. Wesley assigned the leadership of both classes and bands to ordinary members of the societies, but he carefully regulated their activities through supervision and detailed rules.

The classes provided support and discipline. The symbol of discipline was the renewable ticket with which class members could secure admission to the meetings. Members who failed to attend regularly or who fell into transgression lost their tickets. The symbol of support was the class book in which leaders noted the inner "state" of each member. The classes were filled with saints and sinners who were "awakened," or "doubtful," or who claimed to be either "justified" or "perfected in love," and the class leader kept a close watch, with periodic examinations, so that care could be given to each member according to individual needs.[5]

The dialectic of limit and possibility appeared most clearly in the bands, which were designed "to obey that command of God, 'Confess your faults one to another, and pray one for another, that ye may be healed' (Jas. 5: 16)." The bands met at least once a week for singing, prayer, and confession. Fewer than half the early English Methodists participated in the band meetings, and they never caught on in most other countries, but Wesley had high hopes for them. We intend, he wrote, "to speak each of us in order, freely and plainly, the true state of our souls, with the faults we have committed in thought, word, or deed, and the temptations we have felt since our last meeting."[6]

In the band meetings, early Methodists asked each other "as many and as searching questions as may be, concerning their state, sins and temptations." Wesley expected them to want to be told of their faults and to welcome queries and reproofs that "cut to the quick." He thought that they should overcome even any desire to withhold secrets from the group.[7] The intention of such rigorous inquiry was that Methodists might begin to realize the possibility of having the "love of God shed abroad in [their] heart[s]," but that required a confession of the limits imposed by sin, finitude, and temptation. The possibility of love required an acknowledgment of limits; the acceptance of limits became possible through love.[8]

The tone and purposes of the band meetings bear a similarity to the goals espoused in certain forms of modern group therapy. One might speculate that it was the heritage of pietist introspection which inclined so many twentieth-century Methodists to welcome therapeutic groups within their churches. In the eighteenth century, however, the introspection had little to do with therapy and everything to do with piety.

Nevertheless, the societies and classes led to innovative forms of care for the ill even then. From each class Wesley designated visitors, who were similar in his mind to the deacons and deaconesses of the primitive church. Their task was to visit the sick two or three days each week to care for their spiritual and temporal needs.

Of special interest is the way Wesley urged women into this service, partly as a way of challenging the maxim that "women are only to be seen, not heard." Wesley thought such an idea barbaric: "And I know not how any woman of sense and spirit can submit to it. Let all you that have it in your power assert the right, which the God of nature has given to you. Yield not to that vile bondage any longer. You, as well as men, are rational creatures. You, like them, were made in the image of God; you are equally candidates for immortality; you too are called of God, as you have time, 'to do good unto all men.'"[9]

He gave his visitors only four rules. They were to be plain and open in their dealings; they were to be mild, tender, and patient; they were to be clean in all they did for the sick; and they were not to be "nice," or fastidious, in the presence of the smells and sounds of sickness. Care required something other than fastidiousness, whether physical or spiritual. He expected his visitors to care for "all that are in a state of affliction, whether of mind or body; and that, whether they are good or bad, whether they fear God or not."[10]

Wesley recognized that the deepest healing often occurred within the healer. Visiting the sick became in his eyes a "means of grace," an "excellent means of increasing your thankfulness to God, who saves you from this pain and sickness, and continues your health and strength; as well as of increasing your sympathy with the afflicted, your benevolence, and all social affections." But the healing of the healer could happen only if the healer were willing to "be present" with the unhealthy, to stand physically and emotionally with them.[11]

Apart from that requirement of "presence," Wesley offered few suggestions to his healers. He thought it was useful to begin with inquiries about external needs—food and clothing—and then to inquire into deeper matters of the soul. But the main requirement was that healers acknowledge their own insufficiency. They were not to assume that their words brought healing, solved problems, or removed pain. They were to do what they could do and then rely on a "strength" outside themselves. Wesley inaugurated his program of visitation in 1741. By 1748 he could claim that through such communal care "many lives have been saved, many sicknesses healed, much pain and want prevented or removed."[12]

In the eighteenth century, Protestant clergy disagreed about methods of spiritual care, and the disagreements divided them into two groups. One group insisted on the need for an agonizing crisis of rebirth and warned ministers against offering premature comfort to persons humbled by that crisis. Such advocates of revivalism as George Whitefield in England and Jonathan Edwards in America argued that sinful souls had to confront fully the awful reality of damnation without being rescued by a premature announcement of the gospel. The sinner had to come face to face with the limits imposed by sinfulness.

A second group denied the necessity of a crisis, insisted on the need for gradual growth in grace, and warned ministers against discouraging the soul and casting it into despair by insisting that it undergo a crisis. Such critics of revivalism as Joseph Butler in England and Alexander Garden in America argued that sinful souls needed rather to hear the promise of the gospel without being subjected to morbid threats of the law. The sinner needed to hear of the possibility offered by grace.[13]

Despite Wesley's convictions about the universality of grace, he was wary of this second group. He believed that one could not expect to cure the sick soul merely by trying "to give comfort." Merely to "preach the gospel" by proclaiming the possibilities of grace was to overlook the need of sinners to recognize the precise "cause" of their condition. And such an oversight was spiritual "quackery."[14]

To discover the cause of spiritual sickness, Wesley thought, the preacher and counselor had to preach the law, insist on rebirth, and probe into the hidden details of sinfulness. Had sin occasioned the spiritual darkness? Which sin? An outward sin? A sin of omission? An inward and hidden sin? Spiritual sloth? Ignorance? If so, ignorance of what? Temptation? If so, what kind of temptation?

Even so, Wesley did not agree fully with the first group either, for he thought that they overstated the human quandary by failing to recognize the universal presence of prevenient grace. His convictions about the need for growth and nurture precluded any exaggerated emphasis on a crisis of rebirth. Drawing on a pietistic evangelicalism and an Anglican sacramental spirituality, Wesley tried, in his reflections on care, to find a balance of caution and comfort, law and grace, limit and possibility.[15]

## LIMIT AND POSSIBILITY REVISITED

Under the influence of revivalist piety, the Methodist tradition gradually permitted the emphasis on conversion experiences to overshadow Wesley's sense of sacramental nurture. Yet the small group, the class meeting, remained the primary setting for spiritual care, and the class leaders maintained Wesley's belief that care required the healer both "to comfort and to exhort." They assumed that the classes would provide both encouragement and oversight, sympathy and discipline. The classes also continued to send forth visitors to the poor and the physically ill, but their main task was spiritual care, and they expressed their convictions in the language of grace and sin.[16]

By the end of the nineteenth century, the balance shifted, as Methodists, along with other Protestants, increasingly insisted that religious care was joyous, not morose; kindly, not ascetic or austere. In keeping with the mood of muscular and optimistic piety in English and American Protestantism, the manuals for class leaders urged that the classes promote "largely a ministry of comfort." Insofar as classes inquired into the inward condition of the soul, they were to exhibit always "the utmost kindness of both spirit and manner." Such a transition naturally elicited complaints: "Probably one of the most marked departures from the old and beneficial features of class meetings," noted one critical observer, "is the lack of directness and point which formerly so generally prevailed." But the complaints failed to deflate the optimism about human nature that began to appear during the 1880s.[17]

The optimism—or, in other words, the diminished sense of sinfulness—paralleled a growing willingness among Methodists in the nineteenth century to revise their conceptions of care in the light of new psychological theories. Even in the early part of the century, Methodist theologians felt drawn toward the popular discipline of "mental science," one of the precursors of modern psychology, which enabled them to isolate and classify the operations of the mind. The mental philosophers sought to understand the differences that distinguished emotions, desires, and volitions; pride, conceit, and vanity; sadness, mournfulness, and grief; fear, dread, and horror; or any other mental phenomena that seemed to mark human thought and behavior. The acceptance of mental science as a discipline auxiliary to theology helped pave the way for the later acceptance of medical psychotherapy as a source of insight into caring.[18]

In the twentieth century, Methodists looked both to the psychology of religion and to psychotherapy for wisdom about care. The psychologists of religion urged pastors to identify the "natural" patterns of religious growth and to recognize that religion was more a matter of attitude and temperament than of intellectual belief. The psychotherapists urged doctors to recognize the therapeutic possibilities inherent in the conscious mind and the subconscious depths within the self. As early as 1905, Methodists began to heed such admonitions. In that year the Boston University School of Theology offered its first course on "The Psychology of the Religious Life and Experience." By 1916 it was offering a course on psychotherapy.[19]

The main impetus for Methodist reflection on the new psychotherapy came from physicians who began in the early twentieth century to explore psychosomatic medicine. A glance at Methodist textbooks in pastoral care reveals the extent of the debt to such early twentieth-century physicians and psychologists as Walter B. Cannon, J. A. Hadfield, and Flanders Dunbar, who investigated the influence of the emotions on mental and physical health.

In the late 1920s, Methodists joined in the new ventures in clinical pastoral education, which exposed theological students to hospital patients and encouraged them to learn from the wisdom available in places of healing. In the following decade, the English Methodist Conference established a Committee on Healing, to help its ministers and laity understand the implications of psychology and psychosomatic medicine for pastoral care. Such programs intensified an interest in defining forms of care that drew on resources from medical practice.

During the 1940s, Methodist churches encouraged clinical programs, seminary courses, hospital chaplaincies, and pastoral counseling centers that could combine the results of medical research and theological reflection. By 1963 in the United States alone, a Methodist Interboard Consultation on Pastoral Counseling Centers oversaw the work of thirty-seven such centers, in which trained counselors sought to reach a deeper understanding of care and caring. In England, the Methodist Society for Medical and Pastoral Practice sponsored conferences throughout the British Isles with the same purpose in view.[20]

In the 1940s, therefore, Methodists appeared to rediscover Wesley's awareness that thoughts and emotions can make people sick. Pastoral theologians took note of the ways that fear, worry, and anxiety seemingly contributed to physical and mental maladies ranging from colitis and hypertension to manic depression. One consequence was a growing interest in the "function" of religious beliefs and symbols.

The pastoral theologians who wrote in the forties seemed at times to advance a functionalist, even utilitarian, conception of Christian doctrine. Carroll Wise observed that religious symbols had no single fixed meaning but could express sadistic, masochistic, or repressive dimensions of the personality. He argued that an adequate conception of Christian care—one that drew on medical wisdom—must embody the insight that religious ideas can serve the cause of either health or illness. Religion, he said, could be a barrier to mental health, or it could promote mental hygiene.[21]

Nevertheless, it would not be consistent with the Methodist tradition to assert that doctrines are to be maintained only because of their functional value. And even if that were a legitimate reason for maintaining doctrines, their functional value cannot always be assumed. The pastoral theologian Robert Leslie has observed that holiness, in the sense of wholeness, is often a condition of healing, but also that "holiness is no guarantee of health."[22]

The postwar Methodist pastoral theologians ran a risk of reducing the tradition to one of its possible functional meanings, but they also recovered Wesleyan themes that earlier Methodists had lost. Their study of psychosomatic medicine reminded them, for instance, that a human being is no dualistic mixture of soul and body but a unified organism, which in its wholeness can appropriately be designated as a soul. Albert Outler has noted that the practical wisdom of the psychotherapeutic traditions has helped Christians recognize again the "interpenetration of the biological and the psychological." To assume that Christian care is merely concern for disembodied spirits is to abandon one of the deeper insights of the Wesleyan heritage.[23]

The awareness of the person as a unity need not lead to any conflict between the pastor, or the Christian layperson, and the trained physician. Methodist pastoral theologians have insisted, again and again, that pastors not confuse their task with the task of the psychiatrist. The therapist cannot do the work of the minister, and the minister cannot replace the therapist.

The local pastor normally deals with immediate needs and questions in a manner that promotes wholeness and stability, but without assuming the duties of the psychiatrist who has the time and the training to work with troubled persons over long periods. By now, of course, some few ministers have themselves received sufficient training and supervision to offer deeper therapeutic guidance. But most of those ministers work in close association with psychiatrists and other physicians. The sense of professional conflict that once precluded cooperation between ministers and physicians has now begun to disappear.

Caring in the Methodist tradition has always borne the purpose of helping other persons grow. Outler has described the "basic substance" of pastoral care in the Wesleyan spirit as a vision of humanity's "incredible journey from the barely human to the truly human to the fully human." But such confidence in the possibilities of growth has sometimes produced an unduly expansive optimism. Pastoral theologians during the 1960s, for example, insisted that "the power of growth can hardly be overestimated" and appealed to the psychologists of self-actualization and self-realization for evidence of such potential. In so doing, they forgot the dialectic of limit and possibility that has marked the wiser moments of Methodist reflection on care.[24]

Even so, when those theologians wrote of a "redemptive force inherent" in the self, they did not necessarily fall into a Pelagian overstatement of human possibility. Rather, they were harvesting the fruit of the Wesleyan notion of prevenient grace. The doctrine of prevenient grace does, in fact, suggest that no person ever stands entirely beyond the reach of some redemptive capacity graciously bestowed.[25]

The tradition insists that such a capacity for growth is a gift that can hardly be understood apart from the awareness of a "context of being and value wider and deeper than can be obtained in the empirical picture of the world."[26] The psychotherapist, like every other healer, works always within a rich texture of presuppositions that normally remain unexplored. The Methodist tradition holds that exploring those presuppositions would lead to the insight that growth requires a trust in the "fundamental reality that creates, undergirds, and sustains all of life."[27]

The acceptance that the therapist can offer a disturbed patient reflects a trust that can itself never be verified and confirmed by empirical proce-dures. The therapist depends finally not on manipulative techniques and methods but on possibilities that are beyond the therapist's power to create. The therapist assumes that healing, rather than sickness, is congruent with the deeper nature of reality; that the capacity for trust, rather than un-remitting distrust, is consistent with the way things are; that efforts to heal are not aberrations in the human community but expressions of its deeper possibilities.

Such assumptions, regardless of how commonplace they might be, are not self-evidently true or even self-explanatory. The Methodist theologian Schubert Ogden has argued that those assumptions, and others, reflect rather "an ineradicable confidence in the final worth of our existence." Such a confidence hints at something "about this experienced whole that calls forth and justifies our original and inescapable trust."[28]

Methodist theologians, then, typically affirm the possibilities of growth, and they ground those possibilities in the deeper reality of God's presence. They do not assume that growth—a conception exceedingly fashionable in the therapeutic culture of the West—is an easy conception to grasp. Words like *growth* are almost empty of meaning when they are used outside a spe-cific tradition that informs their content. Casual talk about growth can imply that the self possesses some potential structure which will simply fulfill itself. But it makes sense to talk about growth only as a concrete process within a historical tradition.

One can speak of Christian growth, or Buddhist growth, or growth ac-cording to the canons of middle-class society in the English suburbs, but we have no universally accepted norm of appropriate growth. For that reason, it is useful always to be specific when one describes the growth that care can supposedly engender. In the Methodist tradition, one can be spe-cific only by using such words as love, faith, and hope.

In seeking ways to engender that growth, Methodist pastoral theologians have looked not only to the Christian past but also to the medical commu-nity. One of the earliest lessons they learned, or perhaps re-learned, was the importance of what Russell Dicks called the "art of listening." Dicks meant a form of listening that included trust, the withholding of censori-ous judgments, and a willingness to follow the leads provided by the other person.

Intrigued with the notion of "directed listening," Dicks urged those who ministered to the sick to listen to them in such a way as to permit their own inner direction and resources to emerge. He believed that such listening was more likely to occur if both the listener and the patient concentrated on the presence of a "third" reality—a common goal, for example, or a project or interest that drew them both beyond themselves. He suggested that every conversation should proceed as if a "third person" were present, someone or something greater than the immediate concerns of the two persons engaged in the conversation.[29]

Dicks's reflections on listening stimulated interest among Methodist pastoral theologians in both England and America. By the early 1960s, pastoral writers were closely following research in psychotherapy which suggested that skillful listening, conducted without judgmental condemnation or the offering of well-meant advice, could seemingly permit men and women to assume direction of their lives and realize fresh possibilities. Reginald Brighton, a member of the English Methodist Committee on Healing, was in 1962 suggesting that ministers could find in the new research on listening a way to overcome the stereotype of clerical counseling as "moralistic, authoritarian, dogmatic, and judgemental." He distinguished between spiritual direction, in which the goal had already been chosen by a person with a religious end in view, and counseling, in which the seeker brought not a goal but a problem to the minister. Brighton suggested that caring for a person with such open-ended problems might well require a willingness to listen and clarify more than an eagerness to provide direction.[30]

The new interest in listening skills grew partly out of the programs in clinical pastoral education that studied clerical effectiveness in hospital settings; it also grew out of research conducted in medical and psychological clinics. But a third source was a recognition that caring for another often required, above all, a readiness to attend to unexpressed feelings. If the counselor were dealing with deep and often irrational feelings as well as with explicit ideas and conceptions, then rational explanations and advice would usually miss the point.

Such a conception of listening proved attractive among Methodists. One reason was that the Methodists had always been deeply conscious of emotions and dispositions. A proposal about listening that sought to penetrate beneath verbal formulation to the deeper feelings underneath had an obvious congruence with the attention to feelings in the pietistic traditions that had influenced Methodist revivalism. Protestant pietists had always insisted that emotional conviction touched deeper springs within the self than did intellectual assent.

Such a conception of listening gave rise to a style of counseling in which pastoral presence with persons in crisis seemed to mean primarily a willingness simply to suffer alongside the other person. That style of caring appeared to be clearly preferable to a triumphal style of caretaking. But Methodist pastoral theologians have also supplemented that depiction of listening with a more active model that encourages an "openness to signs and symbols of the epiphany of God's disclosure in the events of everyday life." In such a style of caring, a counselor joins with another person in the mutual effort to perceive and interpret the clues that might point toward a more hopeful future.[31]

The pietistic heritage encouraged the interest in group therapy that emerged after 1950. Methodist churches had long before abandoned their class meetings and band sessions, but intimate fellowship in small groups remained important. Like the older pietist meetings for devotional purposes, the small groups seemed to offer the possibility of healing and community. Robert Leslie of the Pacific School of Religion has observed that small groups, by providing a way to deal with both individual feelings and interpersonal relationships, provide people a chance both to feel acceptance and to confront limits and boundaries. That kind of group action, he wrote in the early 1950s, could foster "healthy personality growth."[32]

The attraction to small groups as settings for growth reflects a broader interest in the therapeutic possibilities of interpersonal relationships. Some Methodist pastoral theologians have argued that the "deeper, dynamic aspects of personality" are likely to change "only through living relationships which are of a nature that makes growth possible from within."[33] Some, moreover, have displayed a special fondness for therapeutic theories that accent the importance of interpersonal relationships. The American psychiatrist Harry Stack Sullivan, for instance, proved to be especially influential among Methodist theologians in the United States when he promulgated an "interpersonal theory of psychiatry" that stressed the social formation of the self. Their interest in his work resulted partly from clinical judgments about effective medical practice, but it also exhibited religious commitments nurtured by a tradition in which loving relationships within small groups had often provided occasions for profound healing of the spirit, and in which the ideal of loving relationship not only shaped conceptions of healing but also defined the human journey.[34]

Methodist theologians have also warned, however, that human "possibility is not to be so easily attained" as one might suspect from reading popular treatises about positive thinking. The corollary of the Methodist affirmation of possibility is the more sober Wesleyan awareness of limits.[35] Thus the theologians of the tradition have not been hesitant to point out that our resentment of creaturehood, and hence our refusal to accept the limits to our own worth, power, and knowledge, help define the predicament that underlies our need for healing. As the eighteenth-century classes and bands reminded even the strongest Christians of their weaknesses and imperfections, so Methodist theologians today have argued that men and women "must accept and learn to live on the basis of reality rather than on the basis of [their] wishes."[36]

In *Depth Perspectives in Pastoral Work*, the theologian Thomas W. Klink contended that Christian care would rarely prove beneficial without an awareness of inner conflict. Drawing on such theorists as Karl Menninger and Sigmund Freud, Klink suggested that pastoral work often consisted of an unassuming effort to help another person maintain a working fusion of the inner drives toward creativity and destruction, including self-destruction. Such a theory of inner conflict, taken from Freudian sources, may well serve as the therapeutic counterpart to earlier Wesleyan understandings of the tension between a will and understanding pulled in two directions by the power of original sin and the lure of prevenient grace.[37]

A Methodist conception of caring, therefore, will always include the recognition that self-importance can be damaging to one's health. Self-denial, understood as the denial of self-importance, can be the "master key to the right ordering of life," and hence the indispensable requirement for a healing relationship with another person. Albert Outler has suggested that such an interpretation of the human quandary throws unexpected light on counseling. It illumines the temptations of the counselor, who, like every other person, is "human, all too human." It provides a criterion for the diagnosis of particular crises, since it brings a recognition that we are all caught in a similar dilemma. And it encourages a counselor to pay some attention to the moral and spiritual attitudes of the person being counseled. As Russell Dicks insisted throughout his pastoral writings for and about the sick, healing often requires the confession of sins, not necessarily as a verbal exercise but as the willingness to abandon the effort to protect and absolutize the fragile and frightened self.[38]

## CARING INSTITUTIONS

I have used the theme of caring to illustrate the ways that Methodists, especially Methodist pastoral writers, have drawn on medical resources to enrich their understanding of Christian care within the church. The story would remain incomplete, however, without some reference to other forms of caring that demonstrate the interest in health and medicine in the Methodist tradition. The work of one denomination—the United Methodist

Church and its predecessors in the United States—illustrates the variety of caring institutions.

An exhaustive institutional history of caring in the Methodist heritage, for example, would have to accord greater attention to medical missions— to such figures as Lucinda Combs, who went to Peking in 1873 as the first female medical missionary to China and who trained native Christian women as physicians there; or Clara Swain, who during the same period became the first woman physician in India and constructed the first hospital in Asia for women and children. When Swain arrived in India, she immediately established a three-year course in medicine for young women, and at the end of the first three years a medical examining board certified thirteen of her seventeen students for practice "in all ordinary diseases."[39]

Methodists in the United States organized a new mission board in 1844. When they sent the first missionaries to China, the board had one of them —Moses White—prepare for the mission by studying theology at Yale Divinity School and medicine at Yale Medical College. When White arrived in Foochow in 1847, he built the chapel and the dispensary at the same time, and he practiced medicine there until the church could appoint a medical doctor to the post. The early argument for medical missions was that they would prove useful in providing access to the native population; eventually, however, the Methodists, like many other Christian groups, came to view medical missions primarily as a form of service to people in pain. By the mid-twentieth century, they had constructed thirty-nine permanent denominational hospitals in Africa, Asia, and South America.[40]

Much of the support for those early medical missions came from women's missionary societies. Both Combs and Swain, for example, ventured forth under the sponsorship of the Woman's Foreign Missionary Society (1869) of the Methodist Episcopal Church in the United States. The greater part of the funding came not from wealthy philanthropists but from scores of local W.F.M.S. branches which systematically collected small sums, often mere pennies, each week. The popular missionary journals which those women received in return for their support spread throughout the church regular reports about the medical mission. The missionary movement therefore helped to inject issues of health and medicine into Methodist discussions of Christian mission in the world.[41]

The hospitals built by the missionaries now flourish under the leadership of indigenous physicians and administrators. They range from such institutions as the Clara Swain Hospital in Bareilly, India, a teaching institution with fourteen clinical departments training men and women by involving them in the care of its eighty thousand patients each year, to the

Frank S. Beck Clinic in Ancoraimes, Bolivia, a hospital with fourteen beds, a small lab, X-ray, operating, and delivery rooms, a pharmacy, and an out-patient clinic, which charges rural Bolivians about twenty-five cents for consultations and about a dollar a night for in-patient care.[42]

An exhaustive denominational history would also need to include some account of the long history of concern for children with special needs. Wesley hoped to build at Newcastle an "orphan house," modeled after the work of pietists at Halle in Germany, which would feed and educate poor children. His plans never reached full realization, but his brother Charles suggested that George Whitefield build such an institution in Georgia, and Whitefield succeeded in raising sufficient funds for his Bethesda, the oldest orphanage in the United States, which opened in 1740 near Savannah.[43]

The expansion of denominational homes for children in the nineteenth century again coincided with the "emerging voice of the Methodist woman." In the United States, Phoebe Palmer, who directed the Five Points Mission in New York City, skillfully advertised the mission's work with children: James Buckley reported in 1898 that over forty thousand children had received aid there. By the time German-speaking Methodists in America founded the German Methodist Orphan Asylum in Ohio in 1864, women's benevolence societies had been active in the nation for over half a century, and Methodist women assumed much of the initiative in the formation of the children's homes. By no accident, it was Ellen Verner Simpson, the wife of a powerful bishop, who helped organize the forces to build the best-known of the nineteenth-century Methodist homes for children, the Methodist Episcopal Orphanage of Philadelphia.[44]

By the mid-twentieth century, Methodists in the United States operated some sixty-five child-care facilities. They moved away from the permanent, custodial housing of children, transforming most of the institutions into treatment centers with emphasis on short-term treatment and the placement of children in supervised foster homes. The Health and Welfare Division of the Board of Global Missions in the United Methodist Church, for example, works closely with the seventy-five denominational hospitals in the United States to provide hospital services for physically abused or neglected children. The church also devotes increasing resources to the creation of child-care centers which cooperate closely with community health services. By the 1980s, Methodists labored in such facilities in thirty-two countries, providing foster care, feeding programs, and clinics in local churches. They represent another dimension of what caring has meant for the Methodist churches.[45]

A thorough institutional history would also include some attention to the growth of hospital chaplaincies. Not until 1868 did Methodists in the United States authorize their bishops to appoint chaplains to hospitals, and for years the chaplain's ward languished in the shadows of the Methodist system of appointing its ministers. Only after Methodists joined wholeheartedly in the movement for clinical pastoral education in the early twentieth century did the hospital chaplain begin to assume leadership in the church.

A recent study has suggested that Methodist chaplains have increasingly defined their ministry of care with the metaphor of "presence." One chaplain in the study contended that the chaplaincy might well become the agency through which the larger church could learn to "realize more fully the importance of 'being with' those to whom we minister." "There is," he added, "no substitute for frequent, caring presence." The chaplains in that study also revealed, however, an intense awareness of the difficult dilemmas of medical ethics. They spoke about the problems of medical experimentation and transplants, about the moral dilemmas of helping families make decisions about removing loved ones from life-support devices, and about counseling with families and doctors regarding the use of drugs that would hasten a patient's death. They enriched the metaphor of presence by probing its moral dimensions, thereby affirming that such moral concern was itself an essential part of caring.[46]

An institutional chronicle of caring would provide some insight, moreover, into the emergence of hospice care as a form of ministry to the dying. Hospice care can embrace both in-patients and out-patients. The first choice is to provide such care in the patient's own home, but in any case the purpose is to diminish the pain and helplessness of death. Inaugurated primarily by English physicians, the hospice program emerged in the United States in 1974 under the leadership of a United Methodist chaplain, Edward F. Dobihal, at the Yale–New Haven Hospital in New Haven, Connecticut.[47]

The United Methodist Church now sponsors at least thirty-two hospice facilities, and many of the church's hospitals provide additional hospice care. The purpose is to help patient and family retain control of as many decisions and tasks as they can manage; to permit the patient to decide when to discontinue drastic life-prolonging interventions; to focus care on the relief of pain, for both patient and family; to ensure professional care by trained physicians, nurses, social workers, and ministers; and to perform those ministries of care within an environment as homelike and comfortable as possible.[48]

A history of caring by Methodist churches would include, further, at least a glance at relief programs for persons made homeless or hungry by disaster and famine. By 1984, the United Methodists were budgeting almost $13 million a year for food, disaster relief, and the care of refugees in eighty countries. They were spending over $4 million a year to support agricultural projects in Africa, where millions faced hunger and starvation. Seeking out and supporting grass-roots leaders, the Methodists, like other large Christian denominations, worked especially to provide seed money for small-scale projects which promised to help the hungry grow sufficient food without abandoning their homes.[49]

Institutional caring also took less dramatic forms. In 1963, for example, Alan Walker of the Central Methodist Mission in Sydney, Australia, recognized the pain and suffering caused by loneliness. As a result, he founded a telephone ministry called Life Line, designed simply to provide a place where lonely and suffering people could find someone to listen. After several studies revealed the physical and emotional consequences of loneliness, other Methodists expanded Walker's program. In the United States alone, lay men and women, who have received fifty hours of training, answer the telephone at any hour of the day or night in over a hundred locations. The ministry, simply called Contact, represents another form of caring for both physical and emotional needs.[50]

An institutional history of caring would need, above all, to attend to the multitude of ways that local congregations have maintained unheralded forms of care for people in their communities. It would have to chronicle the numberless soup kitchens and night shelters for the homeless; the efforts to include disabled persons within caring communities; the creation of shelters for abused women and children; the outreach to people in prisons; the counseling and support for persons whose marriages are collapsing; the small groups of laypersons who visit the sick and elderly; and the numerous other forms of care which endure because local institutions keep them alive.

To devote part of such a book as this one to those institutional achievements is to run a risk of denominational triumphalism, an error of the spirit to which the Methodist tradition has more than once fallen prey. To overlook such achievements, however, is to neglect an important part of what caring has meant in the Methodist tradition. Obviously they are by no means distinctive Methodist accomplishments; other traditions —both within and without the boundaries of the Christian Church— could point to similar causes and commitments. But insofar as they do reveal some of the enduring impulses within the tradition, they clearly belong in any narrative on Methodist attitudes toward health and medicine.

## WELL-BEING

In drawing on the resources of therapeutic medicine to refine its conceptions of caring, the Methodist tradition has not assumed that health and well-being were mere equivalents. While Methodist theologians have often insisted that health was a part of well-being, an adequate conception of well-being seemed to require an appeal to theological and ethical convictions that embraced a wider range of human experience than did the categories of health and healing.

In the Methodist traditions, the appeal to theological convictions has always suggested that well-being was to be defined not as a state or condition but as a movement, a direction, a process. It implied not a destination attained but a direction maintained, not the ending of a process but the faithful continuation of it.

Well-being within the Methodist tradition is an orientation of the self, defined most simply as the capacity to love. Such a capacity is not understood as a therapeutic achievement, even though therapeutic care can often enhance it. The capacity to love, as Methodists have understood it, is rather a gift, made possible by the life, death, and resurrection of Jesus and sustained by the ethical and spiritual wisdom bequeathed by the larger Christian past. In making that claim, most Methodists do not insist that Christians alone possess the capacity to love God and neighbor. They confess only that their own capacity to love God and neighbor, in whatever degree they find such a capacity in themselves, came not as the result of their accomplishments but as a gift. The Methodist view of well-being must therefore be defined theologically. In fact, most Methodist theologians would argue that a theological analysis of well-being is necessary even for an adequate understanding of our suppositions and presuppositions about health and medicine.

Why, for instance, do we consider health to be good and illness to be bad? The commonsense reply would be that good health brings pleasure and poor health brings pain, and such a reply would be accurate as far as it goes. But it does not go very far. Some forms of illness, after all, bring their own distinctive kinds of pleasure. There are varieties of mental illness in which, so far as one can tell, the patient dwells within a fantasy world that permits no pain to enter. Cure of the illness would mean that the patient would once again have to face consciously the reality of pain. Nonetheless, we do not hesitate to seek healing, even when the healing would reintroduce the pain. If the valuing of health were simply the reflection of a desire for pleasure, our efforts to heal would, in this instance, seem perverse.

Why, then, do we assume that health, which might bring pain, is preferable always to illness, even to illness which immerses its victims in an imaginary world to which no pain can find entrance?

A further commonsense reply to the question would be that good health brings a capacity for social usefulness and poor health imposes burdens on the larger social order. Such a reply, again, would be accurate as far as it goes, and public officials often rightly make decisions about the health of a citizenry on the basis of social calculation. Indeed, the religious traditions themselves have often asserted that one of the values implicit in health is the possibility of loving service to others.

But a closer examination of our presuppositions about health would reveal, I think, that we do not consider health to be good simply because we find it socially useful. There are varieties of personality disorder, for instance, which, when judged from a strictly utilitarian perspective, would seem to enhance a person's social utility. Inner compulsions that drive persons to expend their lives in unrelenting labor, for instance, might well contribute to both the economic productivity and the social well-being of the larger group. And yet we can recognize that the compulsive labor is the result of a personality disorder, and we assume that even the personality disorder which produces socially useful results is still a disorder. We feel obliged, for some reason, to offer healing to the driven even when their drivenness is socially useful.

The truth seems to be that we value good health for other than hedonistic or utilitarian reasons alone. We assume that the disorder of illness is to be overcome even when the illness brings pleasure or produces socially useful benefits. The Methodist would claim that we make such an assumption because we presuppose that the disorder of illness is not congruent with the way things really are. We presuppose, in short, a doctrine of creation.

Our conceptions of health are thus built upon unstated assumptions about the creation. They presuppose the existence of an order, and they also presuppose that the order is to be valued. They assume that the disorder which we call illness is truly incompatible with some deeper order which provides a norm for human well-being. They assume that illness, even pleasant and useful illness, is not the natural or desirable pattern of things. And such assumptions point toward the truths embedded in the poetic Christian doctrine of creation: "And God saw everything that he had made, and behold, it was very good" (Genesis 1:31).

If the doctrine of creation provides a larger context of metaphorical insight that helps us understand why we value health and well-being, the doctrine of the Fall helps us understand the dangers implicit in that evaluation. The doctrine of the Fall is not a journalistic report of an event in the past but a recognition of disorder and an assertion that disorder is not a good. To the extent that illness reflects that disorder, the doctrine of the Fall enables us to assert that illness contradicts the deeper order which is presupposed by the concept of disorder. To the extent that illness results from the greed that prompts businesses and governments to destroy the environment with pollutants and contaminate food with dangerous chemicals, the doctrine of the Fall provides a way of interpreting the forces that subvert the wider possibilities of health.

The doctrine of the Fall also reminds us that certain forms of health-seeking can themselves stand in conflict with well-being. A compulsive health-seeking can take the form of an idolatrous attempt to secure an isolated escape from our common fallenness and finitude. The absolutizing of health can thus contradict the affirmation that well-being is greater than healthiness. When the quest for health subverts the capacity for love, then the pilgrim has gone astray. The doctrine of the Fall stands as a marker along the road, reminding us that the possibilities of straying are always a danger to the larger well-being which defines the journey.

The doctrine of grace also has provided Methodist theologians a way of clarifying the relationship between health and well-being. The Wesleyan doctrine of prevenient grace refers to the gift through which human beings can recognize the distinction between good and evil, harmony and disharmony, order and disorder, and can then move toward the good, the harmonious, the orderly. The doctrine suggests that human life is graced with an impulse toward well-being, which includes a movement toward health and healing. In the Methodist tradition, any movement toward health that implicitly enhances the capacity to love God and the neighbor in service to Christ has been seen as a gracious gift.

The tradition has recognized that the movement toward well-being can lead through the valley of inner turbulence and pain. The doctrine of prevenient grace became a means of interpreting the pain of the inner struggle that often marks the Christian journey toward well-being. The doctrine did not assume that the gift of prevenient grace entailed a smooth movement of body and mind toward health and healing. It assumed rather that the journey toward well-being can sometimes disrupt the organism's movement toward health. The tradition has almost always assumed that the gift of prevenient grace could initiate a conflict between God's gracious call into the future and the soul's recalcitrant yearning for safety and security, and that the inner conflict between the pull of grace and the tug of sinful impulse can subvert physical and mental health.

Far from invariably promoting healthiness, religious depth can lead to periods of agony and turbulence, to dark nights of the soul and pain of the spirit. Once again, then, the theological analysis accents the distinction between health and well-being. Yet insofar as a certain minimum of health is necessary for the larger well-being, then health itself can be seen as the expression of a prevenient grace that points beyond itself to something greater.

Such theological themes guide the Christian journey and define the relationship between well-being and health. Yet the journey itself receives its meaning only from the assertion that human well-being is defined by the love embodied in the life, death, and resurrection of Jesus of Nazareth. The Freudian psychoanalytic traditions have often insisted that human health must be defined modestly as the simple capacity to love and to work. In a somewhat similar manner, the Methodist tradition has insisted that human well-being is defined primarily as the capacity to love and to serve.

Such an insistence offers a useful way of describing the relation between well-being and health. Insofar as health and the quest for health enhance and deepen the ability to love and to serve God and the neighbor, they enhance also the larger well-being which defines the Christian journey. Insofar as health and the quest for health subvert the ability to love and to serve, they subvert that well-being.

Theological insights have functioned in the Methodist tradition to define boundaries, especially the boundaries of the way of love. Well-being, according to Methodists, is a movement defined by dualities: happiness and holiness, penalty and promise, love and law, responsibility and restraint, limit and possibility. The duality helps to mark the boundaries of the way.

To lose the balance of this duality, Wesley thought, was to lose one's way. To sever happiness from holiness would be to fall into a simplistic eudaemonism or a severe asceticism. To emphasize penalty without promise would lead to despair; to accent promise without penalty would lead to a sentimental optimism. To isolate love from law would produce either a loveless legalism or an inner purity of motive without concrete guidance. To propose restraints without responsibility would create a morality of repression; to call for responsibility without incorporating into it a sense of inner restraint would be futile. To lose the inner dialectic of limit and possibility would be to lose both faith in the future and trust in the past.

In its discussions of healing and health, the Methodist tradition has asserted that healing is always a possibility, even when our possibilities seem exhausted, but that we are always finite creatures embedded within a natural order. The polarity of happiness and holiness has provided a way of affirming that suffering is not the proper end of our existence, but that suffering need not be utterly meaningless. The polarity of penalty and promise has served to push against a despairing view of death as the ultimate absurdity and a sentimental view of death as an ennobling experience. The polarity of love and law has preserved both the Wesleyan accent on the sanctified character and the Wesleyan recognition that the Christian life requires structure and guidance. The polarity of restraint and responsibility has countered both the soft indulgence of a culture intent on self-actualization and the rigid narrowness of a culture intent on the repression of natural vitalities. And the polarity of limit and possibility recognizes both the boundaries of human caring and the promise of growth.

The Methodist tradition, like other traditions, has its own distinctive dangers. It has felt the temptation of moralism and legalism. It has on occasion promoted the self-preoccupation that marks the ambiguous side of its inheritance from pietism. It has frequently fallen prey to the allure of the larger culture and advertised itself as a useful ally in the promotion of superficial cultural values. The honor it has given to the warm heart has sometimes led it to value the empty head. It has not escaped entirely the temptation of a facile optimism which refuses to take tragedy seriously. It has sometimes defined holiness as a possession and used it as a mark of its superiority to other traditions with other emphases. It has on occasion confused health and well-being, suggesting, for example, that abstinence from spirits was the mark of life in the Spirit.

Despite such dangers, the Wesleyan polarities do provide one angle of vision on the promise of well-being. And because Wesley himself had such an intense interest in the relationships between well-being and health, his polarities also offer a measure of insight into the possibilities and limits of medical care, healing, and health. Wesley's vision of human alienation and God's grace, of the journey "from the barely human to the truly human to the fully human" provides an option that can illumine our study of health and healing, suffering and madness, dying and death, sexuality and passages, caring and well-being.[51] In providing that measure of illumination, the tradition prepared a map for a journey, a pilgrimage, toward well-being.

# Notes

**Chapter 1/Wesley and His Tradition**

1. John Wesley, "Preface to the Sermons," *The Works of the Reverend John Wesley, A.M.*, ed. John Emory, 7 vols. (New York: J. Emory and B. Waugh, 1831), 1:xix; Wesley, "What Is Man?" *Works* 2:405; Wesley, "Advice to the People Called Methodists," *Works* 5:249; Albert Outler, ed., *John Wesley* (New York: Oxford University Press, 1964), pp. 77, 88.
2. Wesley to Mr. Merryweather, 24 January 1760, *Works* 6:760.
3. Wesley, "Sermon LV," *Works* 1:492; see also Wesley, "The Character of a Methodist," *Works* 5:240; Wesley, "A Short History of Methodism," *Works* 5:246.
4. *Journal of the 1972 General Conference of the United Methodist Church* (Nashville: United Methodist Publishing House, 1972), 1:281; Thomas Langford, *Practical Divinity: Theology in the Wesleyan Tradition* (Nashville: Abingdon Press, 1983), p. 261; Rupert E. Davies, *Methodism* (Harmondsworth: Penguin Books, 1963), p. 194.
5. Wesley, "Character of a Methodist," *Works* 5:241.
6. Ibid. See also Wesley, "A Letter to the Rev. Conyers Middleton," *Works* 5:757; Wesley to Mr. Clarke, 10 September 1756, *Works* 7:287.
7. Wesley, "Character of a Methodist," *Works* 5:245.
8. Ibid.
9. "Doctrinal Guidelines," *Journal, United Methodist Church* (*1972*), 2:2018–19.
10. Ibid., p. 1989.
11. Outler, ed., *John Wesley*, pp. 89, 90, 190, 272.
12. Ibid., p. 273.
13. Ibid., p. 227.
14. *Journal, United Methodist Church* (*1972*), 2:2015.
15. Wesley, "Justification by Faith," *Works* 1:50; Wesley, "An Earnest Appeal to Men of Reason and Religion," *Works* 5:12.
16. Wesley, *Journal*, 1 January 1773, *Works* 3:276.
17. Outler, ed., *John Wesley*, pp. 47, 63.
18. Ibid., pp. 10, 64.
19. Ibid., pp. 65–66.
20. Ibid., pp. 353–83.

21. Wesley, "The New Creation," *Works* 2:84–87.
22. Wesley, "Of Evil Angels," *Works* 3:140; Wesley, "Spiritual Worship," *Works* 2:183.
23. Wesley, "On the Gradual Improvement of Natural Philosophy," *Works* 7:465; Wesley, "An Address to the Clergy," *Works* 6:219; Albert Outler, *Theology in the Wesleyan Spirit* (Nashville: Discipleship Resources, 1975), pp. 6–8.
24. Wesley, "The Imperfection of Human Knowledge," *Works* 2:120; see also Wesley, "The Good Steward," *Works* 1:450.
25. Wesley, "Wandering Thoughts," *Works* 1:372; Wesley, "The Fall of Man," *Works* 2:34; Wesley, "Thoughts Upon Necessity," *Works* 6:209.
26. Wesley, "The End of Christ's Coming," *Works* 2:69; Wesley, "The General Deliverance," *Works* 2:50; Wesley, "The Christian's Treasure," *Works* 2:479; Wesley, "The New Birth," *Works* 1:400.
27. Wesley, *Primitive Physick: Or, an Easy and Natural Method of Curing Most Diseases* (Bristol: William Pine, 1768; 1st ed., 1747), p. iii.
28. Wesley, *The Doctrine of Original Sin, According to Scripture, Reason, and Experience, Works* 5:492–669.
29. Wesley, "Original Sin," *Works* 1:395; Wesley, "The New Birth," *Works* 1:400; Outler, *Theology in the Wesleyan Spirit*, p. 34.
30. Wesley, *Primitive Physick*, p. iv.
31. Wesley, "On Temptation," *Works* 2:213–14.
32. Wesley, "On Perfection," *Works* 2:172; Wesley, "The Christian's Treasure," *Works* 2:480.
33. Wesley, *Primitive Physick*, p. xxi.
34. Wesley, "The Fall of Man," *Works* 2:35.
35. Wesley, *Doctrine of Original Sin, Works* 5:493; Wesley, "A Farther Appeal to Men of Reason and Religion," *Works* 5:35.
36. Wesley, "Original Sin," *Works* 1:398.
37. Wesley, "Minutes of Some Late Conversations Between the Rev. Messrs. Wesley and Others," *Works* 5:201.
38. Wesley, "On Working Out Our Own Salvation," *Works* 2:235, 238.
39. Ibid., p. 235.
40. Wesley, "Predestination Calmly Considered," *Works* 6:44; Wesley, "On Divine Providence," *Works* 2:103.
41. Wesley, "On Working Out Our Own Salvation," *Works* 2:235; Wesley, "Salvation by Faith," *Works* 1:16; Outler, *Theology in the Wesleyan Spirit*, p. 52.
42. Wesley, "The New Birth," *Works* 1:399.
43. Wesley, "The Way to the Kingdom," *Works* 1:63.
44. Wesley, "On Working Out Our Own Salvation," *Works* 2:235.
45. Wesley, "On Charity," *Works* 2:284; Wesley, "Advice to the People Called Methodists," *Works* 5:250.
46. Wesley, "On Working Out Our Own Salvation," *Works* 2:235.
47. Outler, ed., *John Wesley*, p. 285.
48. Ibid., p. 287.
49. Wesley, "Christian Perfection," *Works* 1:358.
50. Wesley, *Journal*, 12 May 1759, *Works* 4:23.
51. Wesley, *Primitive Physick*, p. xxi.

52. Wesley, "Earnest Appeal," *Works* 5:5.
53. Wesley, "A Plain Account of Christian Perfection," *Works* 6:515; Wesley, "The Christian's Treasure," *Works* 2:480.
54. Wesley, "On Visiting the Sick," *Works* 2:329–35.
55. Ibid.
56. *Journal, United Methodist Church* (1972), 2:2013.
57. *Journal of the Twenty-Sixth Delegated General Conference of the Methodist Episcopal Church* (1912), ed. Joseph Hingeley (New York: Methodist Book Concern, 1912), p. 624.
58. Earl Kent Brown, "Women of the Word," in *Women in New Worlds*, ed. H. F. Thomas and R. S. Keller (Nashville: Abingdon Press, 1981), pp. 69–87; Wesley, "A Plain Account of the People Called Methodists," *Works* 5:186.
59. Virginia Lieson Brereton, "Preparing Women for the Lord's Work," in *Women in New Worlds*, ed. Thomas and Keller, pp. 178–99.
60. Ibid.
61. Mary Agnes Dougherty, "The Social Gospel According to Phoebe," in *Women in New Worlds*, ed. Thomas and Keller, pp. 200–216; Paul Neff Garber, *The Methodists of Continental Europe* (New York: Methodist Board of Missions, 1949), p. 37; Charles W. Ferguson, *Organizing to Beat the Devil* (Garden City, N.Y.: Doubleday, 1971), p. 340; Jean Miller Schmidt, "Reexamining the Public/Private Split," in *Rethinking Methodist History*, ed. Russell E. Richey and Kenneth E. Rowe (Nashville: United Methodist Publishing House, 1985), p. 81.
62. Albert Outler, *Psychotherapy and the Christian Message* (New York: Harper and Brothers, 1954), pp. 8, 21–30, 45–51, 57–60, 66, 69, 226, 228; E. Brooks Holifield, *A History of Pastoral Care in America: From Salvation to Self-Realization* (Nashville: Abingdon Press, 1983), pp. 326–28.
63. Paul Ramsey, *The Patient as Person* (New Haven: Yale University Press, 1970), p. xiii.
64. Paul Ramsey to E. Brooks Holifield, 6 December 1985; Ramsey, "A Letter to James Gustafson," *Journal of Religious Ethics* 13 (Spring 1985): 73; Ramsey, "A Tribute to the Late Rev. John M. Ramsey," *Mississippi Methodist Advocate* 2, no. 40 (23 March 1949).

## Chapter 2/Healing and Health

1. Wesley, *Journal*, 16 October 1778; 18 May 1772, *Works* 4:499, 373; 16 February 1757, *Works* 3:621.
2. Ibid., 1 June 1764, *Works* 4:181.
3. Ibid., 28 June 1770; 4 January 1774, *Works* 4:332, 406.
4. Wesley to Vincent Perronet, 1748, in John Wesley, *The Letters of the Reverend John Wesley*, ed. John Telford (London: Epworth Press, 1931), 2:307; Wesley, "Plain Account of the People Called Methodists," *Works* 5:187.
5. Wesley, "Plain Account of the People Called Methodists," *Works* 5:187; A. Wesley Hill, *John Wesley Among the Physicians* (London: Epworth Press, 1958), pp. 1–12; Harold Y. Vanderpool, "The Wesleyan-Methodist Tradition," in *Caring*

*and Curing: Health and Medicine in the Western Religious Traditions* (New York: Macmillan, 1986).

6. Wesley, "Plain Account of the People Called Methodists," *Works* 5:187–88; Wesley, *Journal*, 16 January 1748, *Works* 3:414.

7. Wesley, *Primitive Physick*, pp. 37, 100.

8. Hill, *John Wesley Among the Physicians*, pp. 1–12, 26–32.

9. Wesley, *Primitive Physick*, p. xxvii; Wesley, *Journal*, 4 February 1768, *Works* 4:271; Wesley, *Journal*, 9 November 1746, *Works* 3:618; Hill, *John Wesley Among the Physicians*, pp. 86–88.

10. Wesley, *Works* 7:539–40; Wesley, *Journal*, 9 November 1746, *Works* 3:618.

11. Wesley, *Desideratum*, *Works* 7:539–40.

12. Wesley, *Works* 7:548–50, 555–56.

13. Wesley to Christopher Hopper, 20 November 1769, *Works* 6:788.

14. Wesley, *Primitive Physick*, pp. ix, xi, xxiii.

15. Ibid., pp. viii, ix, x, xi.

16. Ibid., ix, x.

17. Ibid., viii, ix.

18. Ibid., p. xv.

19. Ibid., pp. 34, 73, 89, 90, 127.

20. Vanderpool, "Wesleyan-Methodist Tradition," p. 322.

21. Wesley, *Primitive Physick*, p. v.

22. Wesley, "Thoughts on Nervous Disorders," *Works* 6:576.

23. Wesley, "On Redeeming the Time," *Works* 2:295; Wesley, "The More Excellent Way," *Works* 2:268.

24. Wesley, "A Letter to a Friend Concerning Tea," *Works* 6:567–69; Wesley, "Some Remarks on Mr. Hill's 'Farrago Double Distilled,'" *Works* 6:186.

25. Hill, *John Wesley Among the Physicians*, pp. 69–70; Vanderpool, "Wesleyan-Methodist Tradition," p. 326; Wesley to Lady Maxwell, 5 July 1765; 4 June 1767, *Works* 7:19, 21.

26. Louis Rose, *Faith Healing* (Harmondsworth: Penguin Books, 1971), p. 99; Wesley, "An Extract," *Works* 7:555; see also Wesley, "The Use of Money," *Works* 1:442.

27. Wesley to John Smith, 22 March 1748, and Wesley to Thomas Church, 2 February 1745, in Telford, ed., *Letters* 2:136, 210; Wesley, "A Letter to the Right Reverend the Lord Bishop of Gloucester," *Works* 5:447; Wesley, "Letter to Middleton," *Works* 5:734; Wesley, *Journal*, 18 May 1772, *Works* 4:373.

28. Wesley, *Journal*, 4 July 1770, *Works* 4:332–33.

29. Wesley, *Journal*, 1 June 1764; 13 July 1764, *Works* 4:181, 186; Wesley, "Letter to Bishop of Gloucester," *Works* 5:447; Wesley, "Of Good Angels," *Works* 2:137.

30. Wesley to Thomas Church, 17 June 1746, in Telford, ed., *Letters* 2:257–58.

31. Wesley, "Letter to Middleton," *Works* 5:733; Wesley, *Journal*, 27 April 1766, *Works* 4:228; Wesley, *Journal*, 10 March 1742, *Works* 3:246.

32. Wesley, *Journal*, 28 October 1739; 19 March 1741; 19 May 1738; 21 March 1741; 8 May 1741, *Works* 3:156, 206, 69, 209.

33. Wesley, *Journal*, 26 December 1761; 5 October 1781, *Works* 4:112, 552.

34. Cited in Hill, *Wesley Among the Physicians*, p. 22.

35. Wesley, *Primitive Physick*, p. xxi; Wesley, "The Christian's Treasure," *Works* 2:480; Wesley, "Plain Account of Christian Perfection," *Works* 6:515.

36. "A Narrative of an extraordinary Cure, wrought in an instant upon Mrs. Elizabeth Savage," *Arminian Magazine* 5 (1782): 251–57; "A Narrative of the Cure of Susannah Arch," ibid., pp. 312–18.

37. Vinson Synan, ed., *Aspects of Pentecostal-Charismatic Origins* (Plainfield, N.J.: Logos International, 1975), p. 68; W. McDonald and J. E. Searles, *The Life of Rev. John Inskip* (Boston: McDonald and Gill, 1885), p. 280.

38. R. H. Howard, "A Novel Test of the Efficacy of Prayer," *Christian Advocate* 47 (29 August 1872): 273; "The Practical Power of Prayer," *Methodist Recorder* 12 (12 July 1872): 566; "The Prayer Test," *Christian Advocate* 47 (31 October 1872): 348.

39. Paul Gale Chappell, "The Divine Healing Movement in America" (Ph.D. diss., Drew University, 1983), p. 87.

40. Ibid., pp. 104–53.

41. W. F. Hatfield, "A Work of Faith," *Christian Advocate* 47 (3 October 1872): 314; Chappell, "Divine Healing Movement," pp. 158–76.

42. J. M. Buckley, *Faith-Healing: Christian Science and Kindred Phenomena* (New York: Century, 1892), p. 43.

43. Chappell, "Divine Healing Movement," pp. 145–59; Frank Townsend, "Faith Cure," *Christian Advocate* 57 (24 August 1882): 660.

44. R. Kelso Carter, *Divine Healing* (New York: John B. Alden, 1888), pp. 20, 29, 59, 73, 167, 171, 174; R. Kelso Carter, "Standing on the Promises," *The Methodist Hymnal* (Nashville: Methodist Publishing House, 1964), p. 221.

45. Chappell, "Divine Healing Movement," pp. 340–55.

46. Leslie D. Weatherhead, *Psychology, Religion and Healing* (Nashville: Abingdon-Cokesbury, 1951), p. 7; A. K. Weatherhead, *Leslie Weatherhead* (Nashville: Abingdon Press, 1975), p. 99.

47. Weatherhead, *Psychology, Religion and Healing*, p. 226; "Spiritual Healing," *Methodist Recorder* 77 (23 July 1936): 16.

48. A. K. Weatherhead, *Leslie Weatherhead*, p. 156.

49. Ibid., p. 159; Weatherhead, *Psychology, Religion and Healing*, pp. 142–205, 486–87, 492.

50. A. E. Whitham, "Faith Healing," *Methodist Recorder* 77 (16 July 1936): 15; Weatherhead, *Psychology, Religion and Healing*, p. 227.

51. John Crowlesmith, ed., *Religion and Medicine* (London: Epworth Press, 1962) pp. 29, 31.

52. Ibid., pp. 79–81.

53. Ibid., pp. 57, 100, 116–20.

54. Ibid., pp. 59, 104.

55. Walter W. Dwyer, ed., *The Churches' Handbook for Spiritual Healing* (New York: Ascension Press, 1965), p. 7.

56. Ibid., p. 52; Don H. Gross, *The Case for Spiritual Healing* (New York, 1958), cited in Vanderpool, "Wesleyan-Methodist Tradition," p. 343; Frank Stanger, *God's Healing Community* (Nashville: Abingdon Press, 1978), pp. 17, 25, 40–49, 54, 125–34.

57. Dwyer, ed., *Handbook*, p. 52.

58. Ibid., p. 35.

59. Ibid., pp. 31, 39.

60. Oral Roberts, *If You Need Healing Do These Things* (Tulsa: Healing Waters, 1954), p. 36.
61. David Edwin Harrell, Jr., *Oral Roberts: An American Life* (Bloomington: Indiana University Press, 1985), pp. 88, 92, 119, 383.
62. Richard Watson, *Theological Institutes* (Nashville: Publishing House of the Methodist Church, South, 1906; 1st ed., 1823), p. 658; Thomas Jackson, "Memoirs of the Life and Writings of the Rev. Richard Watson," *The Works of the Rev. Richard Watson*, ed. Thomas Jackson (London: John Mason, 1846), 1:312.
63. William Warren Sweet, *The Methodists*, vol. 4 of *Religion on the American Frontier: 1783–1840* (New York: Cooper Square Publishers, 1964), pp. 378, 486, 504.
64. G. S. Rousseau, "John Wesley's *Primitive Physick* (1747)," *Harvard Library Bulletin* 16 (1984): 242–56.
65. Leslie F. Church, *More About the Early Methodist People* (London: Epworth Press, 1949), pp. 35–40, 43.
66. Coke and Asbury, Introduction to *The Family Advisor*, by Henry Wilkins (New York: Methodist Episcopal Church, 1804; 1st ed., 1793), pp. vi–vii.
67. Ibid., pp. vi–vii, 25; Vanderpool, "Wesleyan-Methodist Tradition," pp. 331–32.
68. Richard Allen, *The Life Experience and Gospel Labors of the Rt. Rev. Richard Allen* (Nashville: Abingdon Press, 1960), p. 49.
69. Ibid., p. 62.
70. Albert J. Raboteau, *Slave Religion* (New York: Oxford University Press, 1978), p. 275; R. H. Rivers, *Elements of Moral Philosophy* (Nashville: Publishing House of the Methodist Episcopal Church, South, 1861; 1st ed., 1859), p. 195.
71. "The Medical Profession," *Methodist Quarterly Review* 47 (1865): 111, 112.
72. O. P. Fitzgerald, *Sunset Views* (Nashville: Publishing House of the Methodist Episcopal Church, South, 1900), pp. 269–70.
73. *Journal* (1912), ed. Hingeley, p. 1385.
74. Walter G. Muelder, *Methodism and Society in the Twentieth Century* (Nashville: Abingdon Press, 1961), p. 48.
75. Thomas Price Hughes, "The Gospel of Health," in *The Philanthropy of God* (New York: Funk and Wagnalls, 1889), pp. 273–81; Davies, *Methodism*, p. 148.
76. Church, *More About Early Methodist People*, p. 194; George Mains, *James Monroe Buckley* (Cincinnati: Methodist Book Concern, 1917), p. 199.
77. Mains, *James Monroe Buckley*, p. 200.
78. Ibid., p. 205; Charles Jarrell, *Methodism on the March* (Nashville: Methodist Publishing House, 1924), pp. 229–54.
79. Donald B. Marti, "Rich Methodists: The Rise and Consequences of Lay Philanthropy in the Mid-19th Century," in *Rethinking Methodist History*, ed. Richey and Rowe, pp. 159–66; Matthew Simpson, ed., *Cyclopaedia of Methodism* (Philadelphia: Louis H. Everts, 1881).
80. Charles Jarrell, *Go and Do Thou Likewise* (Nashville: Publishing House of the Methodist Episcopal Church, South, 1929), pp. 44–51; Mains, *James Monroe Buckley*, pp. 200–201.
81. Mains, *James Monroe Buckley*, pp. 201, 205; Jarrell, *Methodism on the March*, p. 246.
82. *Journal*, Methodist Episcopal Church (1912), ed. Hingeley, pp. 624–25; Jarrell,

*Methodism on the March*, pp. 229, 246; James Monroe Buckley, *A History of Methodism in the United States*, 2 vols. (New York: Harper and Brothers, 1898), 2:431.

83. Jarrell, *Methodism on the March*, p. 246.
84. Ibid., p. 244.
85. Jarrell, *Go and Do Thou Likewise*, pp. 44–45; Jarrell, *Methodism on the March*, p. 245; Buckley, *History of Methodism* 2:432.
86. Susan Carroll, "Task Force 'Strikes Deal,' Recommends Hospital Sale," *United Methodist Reporter* 131 (25 January 1985): 1; see also *United Methodist Reporter* 131 (18 January 1985): 3.
87. "Healing Mission in Battersea," *Methodist Recorder* 77 (10 September 1936): 10; Richard C. Cabot and Russell L. Dicks, *The Art of Ministering to the Sick* (New York: Macmillan, 1936), pp. 16, 37, 74, 96, 117–18, 130.
88. Russell Dicks, *Who Is My Patient?* (New York: Macmillan, 1941), pp. 9–10, 19; Dicks and Cabot, *Art of Ministering*, pp. 16, 37, 117–18; Russell Dicks, *Your Self and Health* (New York: Harper and Brothers, 1939), p. 37; Russell Dicks, *And Ye Visited Me* (New York: Harper and Brothers, 1939), p. 235; Russell Dicks, *Toward Health and Wholeness* (New York: Macmillan, 1960), p. 2; Russell Dicks, *Meditations for the Sick* (New York: Willett, Clark, 1937), p. 26.
89. C. Edward Barker, "Faith in Healing," *London Quarterly and Holborn Review* 176 (January 1951): 43, 49.
90. Carroll A. Wise, *Religion in Illness and Health* (New York: Harper and Brothers, 1942), p. 122.
91. Ibid., pp. 137, 144.
92. Crowlesmith, ed., *Religion and Medicine*, pp. 86, 91, 102.
93. Ramsey, *Patient as Person*, p. 123.

## Chapter 3/Suffering

1. Wesley to Alexander Knox, August 1778, *Letters*, ed. Telford, p. 317, cited in Hill, *John Wesley Among the Physicians*, p. 132.
2. Wesley to Mary Bishop, 1 September 1771, *Works* 7:163; Wesley to Mary Bishop, 15 March 1777, *Works* 7:241.
3. Outler, *Theology in the Wesleyan Spirit*, p. 81; Wesley, "God's Love to Fallen Man," *Works* 2:43; Wesley, "Spiritual Worship," *Works* 2:183.
4. Wesley to Lady Maxwell, 29 April 1765, *Letters*, ed. Telford, 5:134.
5. Wesley, "Letter to Middleton," *Works* 5:754; Wesley, "On Patience," *Works* 2:219–20.
6. Wesley, "Sermon LXXXVII, On Temptation," *Works* 2:217.
7. Wesley, "Queries Respecting the Methodists," *Works* 7:482; Wesley, "The Nature of Enthusiasm," *Works* 1:329, 331; Wesley, "Farther Appeal to Men of Reason and Religion," *Works* 5:93; Wesley, "Awake Thou That Sleepest," *Works* 1:32.
8. Wesley, "Wandering Thoughts," *Works* 1:372; Wesley, "Heaviness Through Manifold Temptations," *Works* 1:421.
9. Wesley, "Thoughts on Nervous Disorders," *Works* 6:578; Wesley, "Human Life a Dream," *Works* 2:461.

10. Wesley, "Of Evil Angels," *Works* 2:145; Wesley to Miss Bolton, 27 September 1777, *Works* 7:117.
11. Wesley, "Of Evil Angels," *Works* 2:145. See also Wesley, "On Faith," *Works* 2:468.
12. Wesley, "Thoughts on Nervous Disorders," *Works* 6:575.
13. Ibid.; Wesley, "The Education of Children," *Works* 2:310.
14. Wesley, *Primitive Physick*, p. 90; Wesley to Miss Ball, 23 May 1773, *Works* 7:100.
15. Wesley, "Farther Appeal to Men of Reason and Religion," *Works* 5:95; Wesley, *Primitive Physick*, p. 90; Wesley to Lady Maxwell, 17 February 1770, *Works* 7:23.
16. Wesley, "Heaviness Through Temptations," *Works* 1:420.
17. Wise, *Religion in Illness and Health*, pp. xi–xii.
18. Paul B. Maves, ed., *The Church and Mental Health* (New York: Charles Scribner's Sons, 1953), pp. vii, 77–96, 221–30.
19. A. Dudley Ward, *The Social Creed of the Methodist Church* (New York: Abingdon Press, 1965), p. 56; Wade Crawford Barclay, *History of Methodist Missions*, 6 vols. (New York: Board of Missions of the Methodist Church, 1957), 3:82.
20. William K. Quick, "Ministry to Mentally Retarded Adults," *Forward* 2 (December 1981): 1, 5, cited in Jack S. Boozer, *Edge of Ministry: Chaplain Ministry of the United Methodist Church, 1945–1980* (Nashville: Board of Higher Education Ministry, 1984), p. 196.
21. Wesley, "The First Fruits of the Spirit," *Works* 1:69; Wesley, "Thoughts Upon Methodism," *Works* 7:315.
22. Watson, *Theological Institutes*, pp. 57–65, 615, 631.
23. Jackson, "Memoirs of Richard Watson," *Works* 1:384, 386.
24. Albert Taylor Bledsoe, *Theodicy: Or, Vindication of the Divine Glory* (New York: Carlton and Porter, 1856; 1st ed., 1854), pp. 97, 150–75.
25. John Thornton, *Bereaved Parents Consoled*, ed. T. O. Summers (Nashville: Stevenson and Owen, 1855), pp. 73–90; N. Vasant, *Rachel Weeping for Her Children* (New York: Nelson and Phillips, 1876), pp. 49–152.
26. Miner Raymond, *Systematic Theology*, 3 vols. (Cincinnati: Walden and Stowe, 1877–79), 3:34–35.
27. Allen, *Life Experience and Gospel Labors*, p. 76; Langford, *Practical Divinity*, p. 118.
28. Hugh Price Hughes, *Social Christianity* (New York: Funk and Wagnalls, 1889), p. 19; Hughes, *Philanthropy of God*, p. 25.
29. Hughes, *Philanthropy of God*, p. 275.
30. Ibid., p. 18.
31. Charles Wesley, "Jesus, Lover of My Soul," *Methodist Hymnal*, p. 126.
32. Charles Wesley, "A Charge to Keep I Have," *Methodist Hymnal*, p. 150.
33. Borden P. Bowne, *The Principles of Ethics* (New York: American Book Co., 1892), p. 66.
34. See Martin S. Pernick, *A Calculus of Suffering: Pain, Professionalism, and Anesthesia in Nineteenth-Century America* (New York: Columbia University Press, 1985).
35. Edgar Sheffield Brightman, *The Problem of God* (New York: Abingdon Press, 1930), p. 113.

36. Leslie D. Weatherhead, *The Will of God* (Nashville: Abingdon Press, 1972; 1st ed., 1944), pp. 9–19.
37. Ibid., p. 35.
38. Ibid., p. 28.
39. James H. Cone, *God of the Oppressed* (New York: Seabury Press, 1975), p. 175.
40. Ibid., p. 182; James H. Cone, *For My People: Black Theology and the Black Church* (New York: Orbis Books, 1984), p. 204.
41. Cited in Elsa Tamez, "Wesley as Read by the Poor," *The Future of Methodist Theological Traditions*, ed. M. Douglas Meeks (Nashville: Abingdon Press, 1985), pp. 76–77.
42. Edwin Lewis, *A Christian Manifesto* (New York: Abingdon Press, 1934), p. 193; Georgia Harkness, *Understanding the Christian Faith* (Nashville: Abingdon-Cokesbury Press, 1934), p. 193; William Strawson, "The Theology of Healing," in *Religion and Medicine*, ed. Crowlesmith, p. 98.
43. Stanley Hauerwas, Richard Bondi, and David Burrell, *Truthfulness and Tragedy* (Notre Dame: University of Notre Dame Press, 1977), pp. 184–202.
44. Ibid., pp. 147–68.
45. J. Robert Nelson, *Human Life: A Biblical Perspective for Bioethics* (Philadelphia: Fortress Press, 1984), p. 164.
46. Ibid., p. 150.
47. Ibid.

## Chapter 4/Dying and Death

1. Wesley, "Letter to Middleton," *Works* 5:754; Church, *More About Early Methodist People*, p. 754; see also Wesley, "Mourning for the Dead," *Works* 2:550.
2. Wesley, *Journal*, 10 July 1736 and 24 January 1738, *Works* 3:28, 55; letter to Charles Wesley, 27 June 1766, in *The Elusive Mr. Wesley*, ed. Richard P. Heitzenrater, 2 vols. (Nashville: Abingdon Press, 1984), 1:199.
3. Wesley, "Mourning for the Dead," *Works* 2:500–502.
4. Outler, ed., *John Wesley*, p. 89.
5. Wesley, *Doctrine of Original Sin, Works* 5:535, 537; John Taylor, *The Scripture-Doctrine of Original Sin Proposed to Free and Candid Examination* (London: J. Waugh, 1740).
6. Ibid., p. 537; Wesley, "The Way to the Kingdom," *Works* 1:65.
7. Wesley, "The Reward of the Righteous," *Works* 2:341.
8. Wesley, "The Fall of Man," *Works* 2:35.
9. Wesley, "On Discoveries of Faith," *Works* 2:408; Wesley, "The Great Assize," *Works* 1:132; Wesley, "On the Resurrection of the Dead," *Works* 2:507–12; Wesley, "Of Hell," *Works* 2:147.
10. Wesley, "On Love," *Works* 2:147; Wesley, *Journal*, 17 March 1770, 7 November 1771, and 12 September 1765, *Works* 4:219, 323, 361; Wesley, "The Rich Man and Lazarus," *Works* 2:417; Wesley, *Journal*, 28 January 1738, *Works* 3:52.
11. Watson, *Theological Institutes*, pp. 383, 390, 615.
12. Bradford K. Pierce, *The Eminent Dead*, introd. Abel Stevens (Boston: Charles H. Pierce, 1852), pp. 350–64.

13. Stevens, Introduction to *The Eminent Dead*, by Bradford K. Pierce, pp. ix–x.
14. John Ffirth, *The Experience and Gospel Labours of the Rev. Benjamin Abbott* (Philadelphia: Solomon Conrad, 1809), p. 197.
15. Thornton, *Bereaved Parents*, pp. 11–110.
16. W. B. Pope, *A Compendium of Christian Theology*, 2nd ed., 3 vols. (New York: Phillips and Hunt, 1881), 1:38; 2:371, 374–75.
17. "Last Words of the Dying," *Christian Advocate* 57 (26 January 1882): 529; "Quietness in Sickness," *Christian Advocate* 57 (26 January 1882): 55.
18. John Abbot, "The Christian in Heaven," *Christian Advocate* 48 (28 August 1873): 274.
19. S. L. Fancher, "Shall We Know One Another Over There?" *Christian Advocate* 48 (April 1873): 121.
20. Maldwyn Edwards, *Methodism and England* (London: Epworth Press, 1943), pp. 78–81.
21. Church, *More About Early Methodist People*, p. 253; James J. Farrell, *Inventing the American Way of Death, 1830–1920* (Philadelphia: Temple University Press, 1980), pp. 94–95.
22. Thomas Ralston, *Elements of Divinity* (Nashville: A. H. Redford, 1871; 1st ed., 1848), pp. 474–91.
23. John Miley, *Systematic Theology*, 2 vols. (New York: Methodist Book Concern, 1894), 2:95, 429, 474.
24. Albert C. Knudson, *The Doctrine of Redemption* (New York: Abingdon-Cokesbury Press, 1933), pp. 475, 496; Harkness, *Understanding the Christian Faith*, p. 143.
25. Herbert E. Stotts and Paul Deats, Jr., *Methodism and Society: Guidelines for Strategy* (Nashville: Abingdon Press, 1962), pp. 324, 331.
26. Dicks and Cabot, *Art of Ministering*, p. 181.
27. Russell Dicks and Thomas S. Kepler, *And Peace at Last* (Philadelphia: Westminister Press, 1953), p. 6; see also Dicks, *Who Is My Patient?* p. 49.
28. Paul Johnson, *Psychology of Pastoral Care* (Nashville: Abingdon Press, 1953), pp. 233–35.
29. Charles V. Gerkin, *Crisis Experience in Modern Life* (Nashville: Abingdon Press, 1979) pp. 74–109.
30. Elisabeth Kübler-Ross, *On Death and Dying* (New York: Macmillan, 1969).
31. Stanley Hauerwas, *Vision and Virtue* (Notre Dame: University of Notre Dame Press, 1981), pp. 177, 181.
32. Gerkin, *Crisis Experience in Modern Life*, p. 96.
33. Wesley, "Thoughts on Suicide," *Works* 7:462–63.
34. Henry Bidleman Bascom, *Lectures on Mental and Moral Philosophy* (Nashville: Publishing House of the Methodist Episcopal Church, South, 1893), pp. 240–41.
35. James T. Laney, "Ethics and Death," in *Perspectives on Death*, ed. Liston Mills (Nashville: Abingdon Press, 1969), p. 250.
36. Ibid., p. 251.
37. Harmon L. Smith, *Ethics and the New Medicine* (Nashville: Abingdon Press, 1970), p. 148.
38. Ibid., p. 166.

39. Laney, "Ethics and Death," in *Perspectives on Death*, ed. Mills, p. 247; Ramsey, *Patient as Person*, p. 164.
40. Ramsey, *Patient as Person*, p. 151.
41. Ibid., pp. 161–62.
42. *The Book of Discipline of the United Methodist Church 1976* (Nashville: United Methodist Publishing House, 1976), p. 91.
43. Laney, "Ethics and Death," in *Perspectives on Death*, ed. Mills, p. 248.
44. Paul Ramsey, "The Indignity of 'Death with Dignity,'" *Hastings Center Studies* 2 (May 1974): 47–62.

## Chapter 5/Morality and Dignity

1. Wesley, "The Deceitfulness of the Human Heart," *Works* 2:473; Wesley, *Doctrine of Original Sin*, *Works* 5:513.
2. Outler, ed., *John Wesley*, p. 474.
3. Wesley, "The New Creation," *Works* 2:82–87; Wesley, "The General Deliverance," *Works* 2:49–57.
4. Wesley, *Primitive Physick*, pp. lx, xi.
5. Wesley, "The General Deliverance," *Works* 2:54.
6. Wesley, "The New Birth," *Works* 1:400; Wesley, "The General Deliverance," *Works* 2:52; Wesley, *Primitive Physick*, p. ix.
7. Wesley, "The New Creation," *Works* 2:82–87.
8. Outler, ed., *John Wesley*, p. 450; Wesley, "On Working Out Our Own Salvation," *Works* 2:237.
9. Wesley, "On Predestination," *Works* 2:39; Wesley, "On Conscience," *Works* 2:378; Wesley, "The Witness of Our Own Spirit," *Works* 1:101.
10. Outler, ed., *John Wesley*, p. 280.
11. Wesley, "An Israelite Indeed," *Works* 2:274; Wesley, "On Christian Perfection," *Works* 1:357; Outler, ed., *John Wesley*, p. 185.
12. Wesley, "An Israelite Indeed," *Works* 2:278–79.
13. Wesley, "The Original, Nature, Property, and Uses of the Law," *Works* 1:309.
14. Ibid., p. 308; Wesley, "The Witness of Our Own Spirit," *Works* 1:101; Wesley, "Thoughts on Slavery," *Works* 6:292.
15. Wesley, "Upon Our Lord's Sermon on the Mount," *Works* 1:223.
16. Ibid., pp. 180, 202; Wesley, "Thoughts on Slavery," *Works* 6:287, 292.
17. Wesley, "How Far Is It the Duty of a Christian Minister to Preach Politics?" *Works* 6:346.
18. Wesley, "Thoughts on Slavery," *Works* 6:286.
19. Outler, ed., *John Wesley*, p. 179.
20. Watson, *Theological Institutes*, pp. 624–25.
21. Ibid., p. 628; Rivers, *Elements of Moral Philosophy*, p. 27.
22. Watson, *Theological Institutes*, p. 627; Rivers, *Elements of Moral Philosophy*, p. 22; Bascom, *Lectures on Mental and Moral Philosophy*, p. 188.
23. Rivers, *Elements of Moral Philosophy*, pp. 145, 195–98; Watson, *Theological Institutes*, p. 658.

24. Pope, *Compendium of Christian Theology*, 3:180, 182, 185.
25. W. L. Watkinson, "Character," *Wesleyan Methodist Magazine* 123 (1900): 385.
26. John J. Tigert, "Ethics the Science of Duty," *Methodist Review* 48 (1899): 72–83, 902–5.
27. Hughes, *Philanthropy of God*, p. 41.
28. William H. Hunt, "Some Aspects of Settlement Life," *Wesleyan Methodist Magazine* 123 (1900): 760–64.
29. Albert C. Knudson, *The Principles of Christian Ethics* (Nashville: Abingdon-Cokesbury Press, 1943), p. 118.
30. Borden P. Bowne, *Principles of Ethics*, pp. v, 208–9; Borden P. Bowne, *Personalism* (Evanston: Northwestern University Press, 1908), p. 278.
31. Georgia Harkness, *Christian Ethics* (Nashville: Abingdon Press, 1957), p. 36; Stotts and Deats, *Methodism and Society*, p. 75.
32. *The Book of Resolutions of the United Methodist Church* (Nashville: United Methodist Publishing House, 1984), pp. 82, 84, 51.
33. *The Doctrines and Discipline of the Methodist Episcopal Church* (Cincinnati: Jennings and Graham, 1908), p. 468.
34. Wesley, "A Word to a Drunkard," *Works* 6:357; Wesley, "On Reproving Our Neighbor," *Works* 2:92.
35. Wesley, *Primitive Physick*, p. xvii; Wesley, "Thoughts on the Present Scarcity of Provisions," *Works* 6:277; Outler, ed., *John Wesley*, p. 178; Wesley, "Directions Given to the Band Societies," *Works* 5:193.
36. Ivan Blackwell Burnet, "Methodism and Alcohol" (Ph.D. diss., School of Theology at Claremont, 1973), p. 34; Wesley, *Primitive Physick*, p. xv; Wesley, "An Extract from Dr. Cadogan's Dissertation on the Gout," *Works* 7:555; Wesley, "A Letter to the Right Rev., The Lord Bishop of London," *Works* 5:345; Wesley, *Journal*, 9 September 1771, *Works* 6:358.
37. R. Wilberforce Allen, *Methodism and Modern World Problems* (London: Methuen, 1926), pp. 107, 111; Maldwyn Edwards, *After Wesley* (London: Epworth Press, 1935), pp. 132–33.
38. See the proceedings for 1796 and 1812 in vol. 1 of the *Journals of the General Conference of the Methodist Episcopal Church 1796–1836*, 3 vols. (New York: Carlton and Phillips, 1855); Henry Bidleman Bascom, "Address on Temperance," *Posthumous Works*, 3 vols. (Nashville: Publishing House of the Methodist Episcopal Church, South, 1893) 2:311–19; *Journals of the General Conference of the Methodist Episcopal Church 1848–1856*, 3 vols. (New York: Carlton and Porter, 1856), 3:1856.
39. *Journal of the General Conference of the Methodist Episcopal Church* (New York: Carlton and Porter, 1864), p. 265.
40. *The Doctrines and Discipline of the Methodist Episcopal Church* (New York: Phillips and Hunt, 1884), pp. 30–31; see also Allen, *Methodism and World Problems*, pp. 120, 131; Edwards, *Methodism and England*, p. 105.
41. Charles W. Ferguson, *Organizing to Beat the Devil* (Garden City, N.Y.: Doubleday, 1971), pp. 366–67; Mary Earhart, *Frances Willard: From Prayers to Politics* (Chicago: University of Chicago Press, 1944).
42. Ferguson, *Organizing to Beat the Devil*, p. 370.

43. See *Christian Advocate* 47 (26 September 1872): 308; "Alcoholism," *Methodist Message* 60 (April 1956): 19; *Discipline* (1956), p. 705.

44. Stotts and Deats, *Methodism and Society*, p. 333; Burnet, "Methodism and Alcohol," p. 6; *Book of Resolutions*, p. 148.

45. *Journal of the General Conference of the Methodist Episcopal Church*, 2 vols. (Nashville: Methodist Publishing House, 1940), 2:659.

46. *Journal of the 1976 General Conference of the United Methodist Church*, 2 vols. (Nashville: United Methodist Publishing House, 1976), 2:1120.

47. *Book of Resolutions*, pp. 146–47.

48. Howard J. Clinebell, Jr., *Understanding and Counseling the Alcoholic* (Nashville: Abingdon Press, 1968; 1st ed., 1956), pp. 173, 175, 191, 255.

49. Ibid., p. 138.

50. Wesley, "God's Approbation of His Works," *Works* 2:25.

51. Wesley, *Compendium of Natural Philosophy*, *Works* 7:465.

52. Wesley, "Letter to Rutherford," *Works* 7:465; see also Wesley, "The Case of Reason Impartially Considered," *Works* 2:127.

53. Wesley, "Remarks on the Limits of Human Knowledge," *Works* 7:473; Wesley, "Gradual Improvement of Natural Philosophy," *Works* 7:467.

54. Ralston, *Elements of Divinity*, p. 12; "The Progress of Science and its Connection with Scripture," *Quarterly Review of the Methodist Episcopal Church, South* 11 (1857): 49, 55, 57.

55. W. N. Pendleton, "The Parentage of Mankind," *Methodist Quarterly Review* 9 (1955): 324.

56. See the account of the speech in *Methodist Recorder* 11 (26 May 1871): 1.

57. W. H. Dallinger, "Anthropology and Evolution," *Wesleyan Methodist Magazine* 111 (1878): 296–97; W. H. Dallinger, *The Creator* (London, 1887), pp. 79–80; "Two Theories of Man: Evolutionary and Christian," *Wesleyan Methodist Magazine* 108 (1875): 51.

58. Bowne, *Personalism*, pp. 159–216.

59. *Journal* (1968), 2:1266.

60. J. Robert Nelson, *Science and Our Troubled Conscience* (Philadelphia: Fortress Press, 1980), p. 35.

61. Ramsey, *Patient as Person*, p. 2.

62. E. Clinton Gardner, "Ethical Issues in the Testing of New Drugs in Man," *Journal of Drug Issues* 7 (1977): 275–86.

63. Bruce C. Birch and Larry L. Rasmussen, *Bible and Ethics in the Christian Life* (Minneapolis: Augsburg Press, 1976), p. 119.

64. Wesley, "An Israelite Indeed," *Works* 2:277.

65. Rivers, *Elements of Moral Philosophy*, pp. 227–28.

66. Rivers, *Elements of Moral Philosophy*, pp. 227–28, 232.

67. Knudson, *Principles of Christian Ethics*, p. 191.

68. Laney, "Ethics and Death," in *Perspectives on Death*, ed. Mills, pp. 240–45.

69. For a useful analysis of the issue, see James M. Gustafson, "Context Versus Principles: A Misplaced Debate in Christian Ethics," in *New Theology 3*, ed. Martin E. Marty and Dean G. Peerman (New York: Macmillan, 1966), pp. 69–102, and James M. Gustafson, "Christian Ethics and Social Policy," in *Faith and Ethics*,

ed. Paul Ramsey (New York: Harper and Row, 1957), pp. 126–29. Gustafson is not a Methodist, but his analysis is helpful in sorting out issues that have persisted in the Wesleyan tradition for a long time.

## Chapter 6/Passages and Sexuality

1. Wesley, *Explanatory Notes Upon the New Testament* (New York: Lane and Tippet, 1847), p. 147.
2. Ibid., p. 524.
3. Wesley, "On Visiting the Sick," *Works* 2:333; Wesley, "On the Education of Children," *Works* 2:314.
4. Wesley, "On the Education of Children," *Works* 2:311–12.
5. Ibid., pp. 313–14.
6. Ibid., pp. 312–15.
7. Ibid., p. 312.
8. Cited in Philip Greven, *The Protestant Temperament* (New York: Alfred A. Knopf, 1977), p. 36.
9. Ibid., p. 38.
10. Ibid.
11. Wesley, "On Obedience to Parents," *Works* 2:318.
12. Wesley, "A Plain Account of the Kingswood School," *Works* 7:336–44; Wesley, "Remarks on the State of Kingswood School," *Works* 7:344–45.
13. "An Account of an Amour of John Wesley," in *The Elusive Mr. Wesley: John Wesley His Own Biographer*, by Richard P. Heitzenrater, 2 vols. (Nashville: Abingdon Press, 1984) 1:175–84.
14. Ibid.
15. Ibid.
16. Wesley, *Explanatory Notes*, p. 420; Wesley, "Thoughts on a Single Life," *Works* 6:540; Wesley, "A Thought Upon Marriage," *Works* 6:544; Wesley, "The Large Minutes," *Works* 5:217.
17. Wesley, *Explanatory Notes*, p. 22; Wesley, "Thoughts on a Single Life," *Works* 2:542; Wesley "On Redeeming the Time," *Works* 2:297.
18. Wesley, *Explanatory Notes*, p. 420.
19. Wesley, *Explanatory Notes*, p. 420; Wesley, "On Friendship with the World," *Works* 2:199, 203; Wesley, "On Family Religion," *Works* 2:302.
20. Wesley, "On Family Religion," *Works* 2:302–3.
21. V. H. H. Green, *The Young Mr. Wesley* (London: Wyvern Books, 1963; 1st ed., 1961), pp. 26–27.
22. Greven, *The Protestant Temperament*. See also Greven, *Child-Rearing Concepts, 1628–1861: Historical Sources* (Itasca, Ill.: Peacock Publishers, 1973).
23. *Journal*, United Methodist Church (1972), 2:1072.
24. Watson, *Theological Institutes*, pp. 664–65, 666.
25. Ibid.
26. Bascom, *Lectures on Mental and Moral Philosophy*, pp. 225–26; Rivers, *Elements of Moral Philosophy*, pp. 291–99.
27. Watson, *Theological Institutes*, p. 666.

28. Raymond, *Systematic Theology*, 3:171; *Cyclopaedia of Methodism*, ed. Simpson, s.v. "marriage."
29. Bowne, *Principles of Ethics*, p. 232.
30. *Journal*, United Methodist Church (1976), 2:1175.
31. *Journal*, United Methodist Church (1976), 2:1175; *Encyclopedia of World Methodism*, ed. Nolan B. Harmon, 2 vols. (Nashville: Abingdon Press, 1974), s.v. "Ethical Traditions, British Methodism" (E. Rogers); *Journal* (1968), 2:1267. See also Muriel Hopwood and Kenneth Greet, "More to Be Saved?" *Methodist Magazine*, March 1967, pp. 4–7.
32. *Journal of the 1968 General Conference of the United Methodist Church*, 2 vols. (Nashville: United Methodist Publishing House, 1968), 2:1267.
33. Ibid.
34. Wesley, "On Friendship with the World," *Works* 2:203; Bowne, *Principles of Ethics*, p. 239. See also *Cyclopaedia of Methodism*, s.v. "marriage."
35. *Book of Discipline* (1904), para. 66, cited in Muelder, *Methodism and Society in the Twentieth Century*, p. 327.
36. Leonard Brown, "The Methodist Attitude on Divorce and Remarriage," *Methodist Magazine*, June 1961, pp. 207–10.
37. *Journal*, United Methodist Church (1968), 2:1449.
38. "Christian View of Marriage," *Methodist Recorder* 80 (27 July 1939), p. 21.
39. "Declaration on the Christian View of Marriage and the Family," *Statements on Parenthood and the Population Problem*, ed. Richard Fagley (New York and Geneva: World Council of Churches, 1960), p. 24.
40. *Encyclopedia of World Methodism*, s.v. "Ethical Traditions, British Methodism."
41. Fagley, ed., *Statements on Parenthood*, p. 34.
42. *Encyclopedia of World Methodism*, s.v. "Social Concerns, British" (John Kent).
43. *Journal*, United Methodist Church (1976), 2:1164.
44. Knudson, *Principles of Christian Ethics*, p. 209.
45. *Journal*, United Methodist Church (1976), 2:1167.
46. Wesley, "Thoughts on a Single Life," *Works* 6:542.
47. Rivers, *Elements of Moral Philosophy*, p. 292.
48. Weatherhead, *The Mastery of Sex Through Psychology and Religion* (New York: Macmillan, 1932), pp. 124–25.
49. Ibid.; A. K. Weatherhead, *Leslie Weatherhead*, p. 112.
50. Ellis B. Johnson, *Youth Views Sexuality* (Nashville: United Methodist Publishing House, 1971), p. 72; Anne C. Blanchard, *Sexually Speaking—Who Am I?* (Nashville: United Methodist Publishing House, 1973), p. 24.
51. Theodore Jennings, "Homosexuality and the Christian Faith: A Theological Reflection," *Homosexuality and Ethics*, ed. Edward Batchelor, Jr. (New York: Pilgrim Press, 1980), pp. 211–21.
52. *Encyclopedia of World Methodism*, s.v. "Ethical Traditions, British Methodism."
53. Paul Ramsey, "Abortion: A Review Article," *Thomist* 37 (January 1973): 176, 190–94.
54. Albert Outler, "The Beginnings of Personhood: Theological Considerations," *Perkins Journal* 27 (1973): 28–33.
55. *Journal*, United Methodist Church (1976), 2:1164, 1176.
56. Outler, "Beginnings of Personhood," p. 30.

57. Smith, *Ethics and the New Medicine*, p. 52.
58. Outler, "Beginnings of Personhood," p. 32. See also Hauerwas, *Community of Character* (Notre Dame, Ind.: University of Notre Dame Press, 1981), pp. 212–29; E. Clinton Gardner, "Abortion: From the Perspective of Responsibility," *Perkins Journal* 30 (1977): 10–28.
59. Cited in Paul Ramsey, *Three on Abortion*, Child and Family Reprint Booklet Series (Oak Park, Ill.: Child and Family, 1978), p. 62.
60. *Journal*, United Methodist Church (1976), 2:1165.
61. *Journal*, United Methodist Church (1968), 2:1267–68.
62. *Journal*, United Methodist Church (1972), 2:1057; see also *Journal*, United Methodist Church (1976), 2:1176.
63. *Journal*, United Methodist Church (1972), 2:1057.
64. Jarrell, *Methodism on the March*, p. 196.
65. Carroll Wise, *Psychiatry and the Bible* (New York: Harper and Row, 1956), p. 77.
66. *Journal*, United Methodist Church (1976), 2:1169.
67. Wesley, "On Visiting the Sick," *Works* 2:334; Eric McCoy North, *Early Methodist Philanthropy* (New York: Methodist Book Concern, 1914) p. 84.
68. John Thornton, *Solid Resources for Old Age* (London: William Baynes, 1824), pp. 3, 12, 25, 61.
69. Grant Shockley, "The A.M.E. and the A.M.E. Zion Church," *The History of American Methodism*, ed. Emory Stevens Bucke, 3 vols. (Nashville: Abingdon Press, 1964), 2:551; Buckley, *History of Methodism* 2:429; Ralph E. Diffendorfer, ed., *The World Service of the Methodist Episcopal Church* (Chicago: Methodist Book Concern, 1923), p. 602.
70. Paul B. Maves and J. Lennart Cedarleaf, *Older People and the Church* (Nashville: Abingdon-Cokesbury Press, 1949), p. 226.
71. Ibid., pp. 20, 75, 204, 245.
72. Ibid., pp. 239, 245, 252. *Directory of Health and Welfare Ministries* (Dayton, Ohio: United Methodist Association of Health and Welfare Ministries, 1984), pp. 3–26.
73. Maves and Cedarleaf, *Older People and the Church*, pp. 57, 75.
74. Ibid., p. 204.

## Chapter 7/Caring and Well-Being

1. Wesley, "Plain Account of the People Called Methodists," *Works* 5:177, 179, 183.
2. Ibid.
3. Outler, ed., *John Wesley*, p. 180.
4. Carroll A. Wise, "The Pastoral Counselor," *The Pastoral Counselor* 5 (1966): 4–5.
5. David Lowes Watson, "The Origins and Significance of the Early Methodist Class Meeting" (Ph.D. diss., Duke University, 1978), pp. 318–22.
6. Outler, ed., *John Wesley*, pp. 180–181; David Michael Henderson, "John Wesley's Instructional Groups" (Ph.D. diss., Indiana University, 1980), p. 176; Watson, "Early Methodist Class Meeting," p. 363; Frank Baker, *From Wesley to Asbury* (Durham: Duke University Press, 1976), p. 196.
7. Outler, ed., *John Wesley*, pp. 180–81.

8. Ibid.; David Michael Henderson, "John Wesley's Instructional Groups" (Ph.D. diss., Indiana University, 1980), p. 176; Watson, "Early Methodist Class Meeting," p. 363.

9. Wesley, "On Visiting the Sick," *Works* 2:335.

10. Ibid., pp. 330, 331; Wesley, "Plain Account of the People Called Methodists," *Works* 5:187.

11. Wesley. "On Visiting the Sick," *Works* 2:330–31.

12. Ibid., pp. 330, 331; Wesley, "Plain Account of the People Called Methodists," *Works* 5:187.

13. Holifield, *History of Pastoral Care*, pp. 92–93.

14. Wesley, "The Wilderness State," *Works* 1:413–16.

15. Ibid.; Albert Outler, "Pastoral Care in the Wesleyan Spirit," *Perkins Journal* 25 (1971): 4–11.

16. W. L. Prottsman, *The Class-Leader* (St. Louis: Methodist Book Depository, 1856), p. 28; Leonidas Rosser, *Class Meetings* (Richmond: L. Johnson, 1855), pp. 149, 151, 229; Charles Kemp, *Physicians of the Soul* (New York: Macmillan, 1947), pp. 51, 68–84.

17. John Atkinson, *The Class Leader* (New York: Nelson and Phillips, 1874), pp. 67, 154, 205.

18. Holifield, *History of Pastoral Care*, p. 149; Bascom, *Lectures in Mental and Moral Philosophy*, pp. 70–134.

19. Francis Strickland, "Pastoral Psychology: A Retrospect," *Pastoral Psychology* 4 (1953): 9; Kemp, *Physicians of the Soul*, pp. 243–44.

20. Charles A. Van Wagner, "The AAPC: The Formative Years (A History of the American Association of Pastoral Counselors, 1963–1970)" (S.T.D. thesis, Emory University, 1985), p. 44.

21. Wise, *Religion in Illness and Health*, pp. 146, 153.

22. Robert Leslie, *Health, Healing, and Holiness* (Nashville: Methodist Publishing, House, 1971), p. 17.

23. Outler, *Psychotherapy and the Christian Message*, p. 25.

24. Paul E. Johnson, *Personality and Religion* (Nashville: Abingdon Press, 1962), p. 259.

25. Outler, "Pastoral Care in Wesleyan Spirit," p. 10; Johnson, *Personality and Religion*, p. 259; Carroll A. Wise, *Pastoral Counseling: Its Theory and Practice* (New York: Harper and Brothers, 1951), p. 9.

26. Outler, *Psychotherapy and the Christian Message*, p. 129.

27. Wise, *Psychiatry and the Bible*, p. 2.

28. Schubert Ogden, *The Reality of God and Other Essays* (London: SCM Press, 1967; 1st ed., 1963), p. 37.

29. Dicks, *Who Is My Patient?* p. 87; Dicks and Cabot, *Art of Ministering*, pp. 16, 74, 96, 117–18, 190, 197.

30. Reginald Brighton, "Healing and the Minister," in *Religion and Medicine*, ed. Crowlesmith, pp. 153, 155.

31. Gerkin, *Crisis Experience in Modern Life*, pp. 321, 327.

32. Robert Leslie, "Pastoral Group Psychotherapy," in *Journal of Pastoral Care* 6 (1952): 56–61; Robert Leslie, "Growth Through Group Interaction," *Journal of Pastoral Care* 5 (1951): 39.

33. Wise, *Psychiatry and the Bible*, p. x.
34. Holifield, *History of Pastoral Care*, pp. 318, 320; Howard Clinebell, *Mental Health Through Christian Community* (Nashville: Abingdon Press, 1965), p. 24.
35. Outler, *Psychotherapy and the Christian Message*, p. 147; Albert Outler, *A Christian Context for Counseling* (New Haven: Hazen Foundation, 1946), pp. 8–9.
36. Wise, *Psychiatry and the Bible*, p. 20.
37. Thomas Klink, *Depth Perspectives in Pastoral Work* (Philadelphia: Fortress Press, 1965), pp. 17–32.
38. Outler, *Psychotherapy and the Christian Message*, pp. 140, 141, 143; Outler, *Christian Context*, p. 10; Dicks, *Who Is My Patient?* p. 19.
39. *Encyclopedia of World Methodism*, s.v. "Missions and Organized Methodist Missionary Work," (N. B. Harmon); Barclay, *History of Methodist Missions* 3:192.
40. Barclay, *History of Methodist Missions* 3:191–93.
41. Rosemary Skinner Keller, "Creating a Sphere for Women," *Women in New Worlds*, ed. Thomas and Keller, pp. 246–60.
42. Doris Franklin, "The Moving Spirit of Clara Swain," *New World Outlook* 44 (December 1984): 478–81; Natalie Barber, "Treating Patients with Compassion," *New World Outlook* 37 (September 1977): 406–7.
43. See Eric McCoy North, *Early Methodist Philanthropy* (New York: Methodist Book Concern, 1914), pp. 87, 89.
44. Buckley, *History of Methodism* 2:429–30; Keith Melder, "Ladies Bountiful: Organized Women's Benevolence in Early 19th Century America," *New York History* 43 (1967): 231–54; Joanna Bowen Gillespie, "The Emerging Voice of the Methodist Woman," in *Rethinking Methodist History*, ed. Richey and Rowe, pp. 148–58.
45. *Quadrennial Reports, 1972* (Nashville: Methodist Publishing House, 1972), pp. 209, 210; Suzanne Shaughnessy, "Aiding a Million Children," *New World Outlook* 43 (July–August 1983): 313–15.
46. Boozer, *Edge of Ministry*, pp. 131, 171.
47. John Justice, "Hospice Care: Hard and Loving Work," *New World Outlook* 43 (July–August 1983): 316–19.
48. Ibid.
49. Nelson Navarro, "The Greening of Africa," *New World Outlook* 43 (October 1983): 432–35; Sheila Bruton, "Erasing Hurt and Hunger," *New World Outlook* 44 (April–May 1984): 171–74.
50. Dennis R. Gable, "Contact: A Telephone Ministry that Makes a Difference," *New World Outlook* 44 (January 1984): 62–65.
51. Outler, "Pastoral Care in Wesleyan Spirit," p. 10.

# DATE DUE

|  |  |  |  |
|--|--|--|--|
|  |  |  |  |
|  |  |  |  |
|  |  |  |  |
|  |  |  |  |
|  |  |  |  |
|  |  |  |  |
|  |  |  |  |
|  |  |  |  |
|  |  |  |  |
|  |  |  |  |
|  |  |  |  |
|  |  |  |  |
|  |  |  |  |
|  |  |  |  |
|  |  |  |  |
|  |  |  |  |
|  |  |  |  |